Syndromes in Organ Failure

Editor

BENJAMIN A. SMALLHEER

NURSING CLINICS
OF NORTH AMERICA

www.nursing.theclinics.com

Consulting Editor
STEPHEN D. KRAU

September 2018 • Volume 53 • Number 3

ELSEVIER

1600 John F. Kennedy Boulevard • Suite 1800 • Philadelphia, Pennsylvania, 19103-2899

http://www.theclinics.com

NURSING CLINICS OF NORTH AMERICA Volume 53, Number 3
September 2018 ISSN 0029-6465, ISBN-13: 978-0-323-64231-6

Editor: Kerry Holland
Developmental Editor: Casey Potter

Nursing Clinics of North America (ISSN 0029-6465) is published quarterly by Elsevier Inc., 360 Park Avenue South, New York, NY 10010-1710. Months of issue are March, June, September, and December. Periodicals postage paid at New York, NY and additional mailing offices. Subscription price per year is, $155.00 (US individuals), $465.00 (US institutions), $275.00 (international individuals), $567.00 (international institutions), $220.00 (Canadian individuals), $567.00 (Canadian institutions), $100.00 (US students), and $135.00 (international students). To receive student/resident rate, orders must be accompanied by name of affiliated institution, date of term, and the signature of program/residency coordinator on institution letterhead. Orders will be billed at individual rate until proof of status is received. Foreign air speed delivery is included in all *Clinics* subscription prices. All prices are subject to change without notice. **POSTMASTER:** Send address changes to *Nursing Clinics*, Elsevier Health Sciences Division, Subscription Customer Service, 3251 Riverport Lane, Maryland Heights, MO 63043. **Customer Service: Telephone: 1-800-654-2452** (U.S. and Canada); **1-314-447-8871 (outside U.S. and Canada). Fax: 1-314-447-8029. E-mail: journalscustomerservice-usa@elsevier.com** (for print support) and **journalsonlinesupport-usa@elsevier.com** (for online support).

Nursing Clinics of North America is covered in *EMBASE/Excerpta Medica, MEDLINE/PubMed (Index Medicus), Social Sciences Citation Index, Current Contents, ASCA, Cumulative Index to Nursing, RNdex Top 100,* and Allied Health Literature and International Nursing Index (INI).

Contributors

CONSULTING EDITOR

STEPHEN D. KRAU, PhD, RN, CNE
Associate Professor (Retired), Vanderbilt University Medical Center, Vanderbilt University School of Nursing, Nashville, Tennessee

EDITOR

BENJAMIN A. SMALLHEER, PhD, RN, ACNP-BC, FNP-BC, CCRN, CNE
Assistant Professor of Nursing, Lead Faculty, Adult-Gerontology Acute Care Nurse Practitioner Program, Duke University School of Nursing, Durham, North Carolina

AUTHORS

BRITTANY ABELN, BSN, RN
Doctoral Student, The University of Arizona, College of Nursing, Tucson, Arizona

MARGARET J. CARMAN, DNP, ACNP-BC, ENP-BC, FAEN
Program Director, Adult-Gerontology Acute Care Nurse Practitioner Program, Department of Advanced Nursing Practice, Georgetown University School of Nursing & Health Studies, Washington, DC

RICKETTA CLARK, DNP, FNP-BC
Assistant Professor, Nursing, The University of Tennessee Health Science Center, Memphis, Tennessee

SHANNON COLE, DNP, APRN-BC
Vanderbilt University School of Nursing, Nashville, Tennessee

ELIZABETH COMPTON, RN, MSN, AGACNP-BC
Trauma Nurse Practitioner, Division of Trauma and Surgical Critical Care, Vanderbilt University Medical Center, Nashville, Tennessee

KATHRYN D. FUKUMOTO, BSN, RN, CCRN
Registered Nurse, Neurosciences and Trauma Intensive Care Unit, John Muir Medical Center, Walnut Creek, California

LAUREN E. FUKUMOTO, MSN, AGACNP-BC, CNP, CCRN
Nurse Practitioner, Neurosurgery, Mount Carmel Health Systems, Columbus, Ohio

ANGELIKA A. GABRIELSKI, FNP-BC
Nurse Practitioner, Division of Endocrinology, Metabolism and Nutrition, Nursing, Duke University Medical Center, Durham, North Carolina

FELISA B. HAMMONDS, FNP-BC
Duke University School of Nursing, Durham, North Carolina

RAGAN JOHNSON, DNP, FNP-BC
Assistant Professor, Nursing, Duke University School of Nursing, Durham, North Carolina

KATHRYN EVANS KREIDER, DNP, FNP-BC, BC-ADM
Assistant Professor, Lead Faculty, Endocrinology Specialty, Nurse Practitioner and Coordinator for APP's, Division of Endocrinology, Metabolism and Nutrition, Duke University School of Nursing, Duke University Medical Center, Durham, North Carolina

RENE LOVE, PhD, DNP, PMHNP-BC, FNAP, FAANP
DNP Director, Clinical Associate Professor, The University of Arizona, College of Nursing, Tucson, Arizona

RENATE K. MEIER, MS, MSN, WHNP-BC, SANE-A
Assistant Professor, Department of Obstetrics and Gynecology, Vanderbilt University School of Medicine, Vanderbilt University Medical Center, Nashville, Tennessee

BRETT MORGAN, DNP, CRNA
Assistant Professor, Director, Nurse Anesthesia Program to Brett Morgan, Duke University School of Nursing, Nurse Anesthesia Program, Durham, North Carolina

ABBY LUCK PARISH, DNP, AGPCNP-BC, GNP-BC, FNAP
Assistant Professor, Vanderbilt University School of Nursing, Nashville, Tennessee

ANGELA RICHARD-EAGLIN, DNP, MSN, APRN, FNP-BC
Assistant Professor, Healthcare in Adult Populations Division, Duke University School of Nursing, Co-Director, VA Nursing Academic Partnership in Graduate Education Primary Care Residency Program, Durham, North Carolina

SHARRON RUSHTON, DNP, MS, RN, CCM
Assistant Clinical Professor, Duke University School of Nursing, Durham, North Carolina

BENJAMIN A. SMALLHEER, PhD, RN, ACNP-BC, FNP-BC, CCRN, CNE
Assistant Professor of Nursing, Lead Faculty, Adult-Gerontology Acute Care Nurse Practitioner Program, Duke University School of Nursing, Durham, North Carolina

STEVE WOODEN, DNP, CRNA, NSPM
Department of Anesthesia, Wooden Anesthesia PC, Boone County Medical Center, Albion, Nebraska

Contents

Diabetes mellitus and its complications are among the leading causes of organ failure around the world. It is imperative that timely, patient-centered care is provided to avoid microvascular and macrovascular damage. People with well-controlled diabetes can live long and healthy lives through interprofessional management, emphasizing optimal, individualized care.

Autoimmune disorders are a category of diseases in which the immune system attacks healthy cells as a result of a dysfunction of the acquired immune system. Clinical presentation and diagnosis are disease specific and often correspond with the degree of inflammation, as well as the systems involved. Treatment varies based on the specific disease, its stage of presentation, and patient symptoms. The primary goal of treatment is to decrease inflammation, minimize symptoms, and lessen the potential for relapse. Graves disease, Hashimoto thyroiditis, rheumatoid arthritis, Crohn disease, ulcerative colitis, systemic lupus erythematosus, and multiple sclerosis are discussed in this article.

Fat embolisms are fat globules that enter the circulatory system, typically through trauma, that may or may not lead to the development of fat embolism syndrome (FES), a rare and ill-defined diagnosis that can cause multi-organ failure and death. The exact mechanism of FES remains unknown, although several theories support the involvement of inflammatory response activation that contributes to characteristic clinical findings. There is no gold standard for diagnosis of FES, and treatment at this time remains primarily supportive. Early recognition of FES symptoms is the most beneficial nursing intervention for combating this serious disorder.

Management of chronic pain has become a significant challenge for primary care providers, and the population of patients with chronic pain is expected to increase. Common syndromes seen in the primary care setting include myofascial pain syndrome, fibromyalgia, chronic postsurgical pain, complex regional pain syndrome, and painful diabetic neuropathy. This article describes these syndromes and presents current treatment options.

Malabsorption syndrome refers to the inability of the small intestines to absorb certain nutrients and fluids. There are several common associated disorders, which may present with subtle and/or overt symptoms. With subtle symptoms, it is difficult to determine the cause, making diagnosis difficult or even inaccurate. Malabsorption can originate from an immune response, an inflammatory process, or alternation of the small intestines by surgical methods. This article reviews common malabsorption disease processes of the small bowel and the resulting pathophysiology. Diagnostic studies, treatment, and prognosis of various conditions within the malabsorption disease state are discussed.

Munchausen syndrome and Munchausen syndrome by proxy are complex diseases that are difficult to diagnose and treat. To assist in this process, an overview of diagnostic criteria with common characteristics and red flags are discussed, with case studies illustrating identification and diagnosis of these disorders. Treatment options are addressed within the context of each of these complex syndromes. The provider's knowledge of diagnostic criteria and treatment options for Munchausen syndrome and Munchausen syndrome by proxy promotes better outcomes for patients. Without an early diagnosis and intervention, the patient is at high risk for severe complications, including organ failure and mortality.

Adrenal insufficiency (Addison disease) and Cushing syndrome are rare disorders characterized by abnormal secretion of adrenal hormones. All patients with adrenal insufficiency and many with Cushing syndrome require lifelong therapy with the potential to affect the quality of life. Management requires gain of a significant amount of knowledge related to treatment, self-care, and how to react quickly in critical situations. Knowledge deficits related to management may cause patients to become critically ill and may even cause death. Ongoing patient/family teaching is crucial for proper disease management and sustaining the quality of life.

Hypogonadism is a clinical syndrome that results in hormone deficiency in men and women. Primary hypogonadism is caused by gonadal (testicular or ovarian) failure. Secondary hypogonadism is the result of a dysfunction within the hypothalamus and/or pituitary. Diagnosis of hypogonadism requires a comprehensive health history, evaluation of the signs and symptoms, complete physical examination, as well as laboratory and diagnostic testing for both sexes. Hormone replacement is the hallmark of hypogonadism treatment. Restoring and/or maintaining quality of life is a major consideration in the management of patients with hypogonadism.

Renate K. Meier

Polycystic ovary syndrome (PCOS) is a commonly occurring endocrine disorder characterized by hirsutism, anovulation, and polycystic ovaries. Often comorbid with insulin resistance, dyslipidemia, and obesity, it also carries significant risk for the development of cardiovascular and metabolic sequelae, including diabetes and metabolic syndrome. Traditionally, the treatment of patients with PCOS has focused on relief of symptoms. Here, the criteria for the diagnosis of PCOS are reviewed, with an emphasis on the stratification of subtypes by metabolic features. Then treatment options are reviewed according to the management goal: relief of hyperandrogenic symptoms, regulation of menstruation, and restoration of fertility.

Sharron Rushton and Margaret J. Carman

Noncardiac chest pain is an angina-type discomfort without indication of ischemia. Diagnosis can be difficult because of its heterogeneous nature. Classification varies by specialty; gastroenterology uses the terminology gastroesophageal reflux disease related versus non–gastroesophageal reflux disease related. Other disciplines recognize noncardiac chest pain as having gastrointestinal, musculoskeletal, psychiatric, or pulmonary/other as underlying causes. Diagnostics yield a specific cause for effective treatment, which is aimed at the underlying cause, but it is not always possible. Some patients with noncardiac chest pain have comorbidities and ongoing pain that lead to decreased quality of life and continued health care use.

Benjamin A. Smallheer

Restless legs syndrome/Willis-Ekbon disease (RLS/WED) is a common sensorimotor disorder characterized by an irresistible urge to move and is associated with an uncomfortable sensation typically in the lower extremities. Dopaminergic neurotransmission abnormalities, genetics, sleep deprivation, and iron deficiency all play key roles in the pathogenesis of primary RLS. Secondary RLS has been associated with other medical conditions and medication usage. A thorough subjective evaluation and complete neurologic examination are key in the diagnosis of RLS/WED. Treatment includes pharmacologic and nonpharmacologic approaches. Referral to a neurologist or sleep specialist should be considered if initial treatment plans are ineffective.

> Neurodegenerative disorders are progressive, debilitating impairments of neurologic function. Dementia affects cognition and function. Persons with cognitive deficits should undergo a full workup and may be treated with cholinesterase inhibitors and/or memantine. Behavioral and psychological symptoms of dementia may be assessed and treated individually. Parkinson disease is a disorder of movement. Levodopa is the standard treatment of dopamine-related movement symptoms. Associated symptoms should be assessed and treated. Other neurodegenerative syndromes are less common but highly debilitating. Currently, there are no curative or disease-modifying therapies for neurodegenerative disorders. Novel therapies or research are in the pipeline.

> Paroxysmal sympathetic hyperactivity (PSH) is a syndrome classified by episodic presentation of abnormal sympathetic and motor symptoms observed in patients with acquired brain injuries. Although the exact physiologic mechanism of PSH is not fully understood, its clinical significance has been well established. PSH diagnosis depends on the identification of symptom presence, severity, and patterns. Treatment of PSH is rooted in pharmacologic management of targeted symptoms. Although recognition and management of PSH is complex, it has meaningful implications on the hospitalization and recovery trajectory for adult patients with traumatic brain injuries.

NURSING CLINICS OF NORTH AMERICA

THE CLINICS ARE AVAILABLE ONLINE!
Access your subscription at:
www.theclinics.com

Preface

Those Conditions You May Not Be Expecting

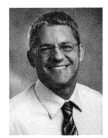

Benjamin A. Smallheer, PhD, RN, ACNP-BC, FNP-BC, CCRN, CNE
Editor

Within our current health care environment, citizens are having increased access to health care and are seeking the expertise of primary care providers for preventative medicine and disease maintenance rather than delaying medical attention until acute care services are required. This shift in patient flow from urgent and emergency settings is increasing the need of the primary care provider not only to conduct comprehensive evaluations focused on wellness but also to assess conditions that may present with vague and unclear causes. Confusing and overlapping disease presentation increases the likelihood of a provider attempting to diagnose and treat, or refer uncommon or "mimicking" conditions for expert consultation.

When considering topics for this issue pertaining to "Syndromes in Organ Failure," I considered my personal perspective as a dual-certified Acute Care NP and Family NP. Often patients are rapidly referred, admitted, and evaluated based on the fear or concern of the "worst possible condition." The reality may exist that the patient has presented with a more unusual diagnosis that could have been worked up in a completely different manner in the primary care setting. It is from this perspective that I felt it appropriate to address a combination of diagnoses: some more often seen in practice along with a few of which are less often encountered. The less common conditions are often a bit more difficult to diagnose and often are a diagnosis of exclusion, yet their identification is vital so that appropriate treatment can be initiated.

It is our hope that this issue of *Nursing Clinics of North America* can serve as a handbook or reference guide when evaluating patients for conditions that may not be as straightforward as the provider has anticipated. We have entertained a variety of body systems and diagnoses encompassing endocrine, immunology, hematology, neurology, gastrointestinal, psych-mental health, gynecology, cardiac, and musculoskeletal. Each article addresses a clinical syndrome that may be encountered in the acute care setting, the primary care setting, or both environments. The authors identify

Nurs Clin N Am 53 (2018) xi–xii
https://doi.org/10.1016/j.cnur.2018.06.001
0029-6465/18/© 2018 Published by Elsevier Inc.

nursing.theclinics.com

the condition, provide relevant background information, and review patient presentation, diagnosis, and current treatment guidelines. Through this, clinicians can quickly and efficiently refer to data and return to the ever-important responsibility of caring for those in our communities.

Benjamin A. Smallheer, PhD, RN, ACNP-BC, FNP-BC, CCRN, CNE
Adult-Gerontology Acute Care Nurse
Practitioner Program
Duke University School of Nursing
307 Trent Drive, DUMC 3322
Durham, NC 27710, USA

E-mail address:
benjamin.smallheer@duke.edu

Hyperglycemia Syndromes

Kathryn Evans Kreider, DNP, FNP-BC, BC-ADM[a],*,
Angelika A. Gabrielski, FNP-BC[b], Felisa B. Hammonds, FNP-BC[c]

KEYWORDS

- Diabetes • Hyperglycemia • Complications of diabetes
- DKA (diabetic ketoacidosis) • HHS (hyperglycemic hyperosmolar state)
- Glycemic control

KEY POINTS

- Diabetes is one of the leading causes of organ failure in the world with high rates of microvascular and macrovascular disease.
- Diabetic ketoacidosis and hyperglycemia hyperosmolar syndrome are two serious complications of diabetes that can lead to significant morbidity and mortality.
- Individualized, patient-centered care is crucial to avoiding complications of diabetes; people with well-controlled diabetes can live long and healthy lives.

INTRODUCTION

Diabetes mellitus (DM) has become a global pandemic. In 2014, it was estimated that more than 422 million people had diabetes worldwide[1] and it is predicted that approximately 592 million people globally will have diabetes by 2035.[2] Additionally, nearly 1.5 million Americans are diagnosed with diabetes every year, and 23.8% of people with diabetes are undiagnosed.[3] The financial burden of diabetes in the United States is approximately $245 billion a year, including direct and indirect costs, a staggering number that continues to climb.[4] In 2014, there were 300 million deaths associated with diabetes and it is the seventh leading cause of death in the United States.[5] Diabetes is one of the leading causes of organ failure, and timely, evidence-based patient education and management is essential to preventing complications.

The authors have no commercial or financial conflicts of interests to disclose. There was no funding source for the production of this work.
[a] Endocrinology Specialty, Division of Endocrinology, Metabolism and Nutrition, Duke University School of Nursing, Duke University Medical Center, 307 Trent Drive, Durham, NC 27710, USA; [b] Division of Endocrinology, Metabolism and Nutrition, Duke University Medical Center, 307 Trent Drive, Durham, NC 27710, USA; [c] Duke University School of Nursing, 307 Trent Drive, Durham, NC 27710, USA
* Corresponding author.
E-mail address: Kathryn.evans@duke.edu

PATHOPHYSIOLOGY OF DIABETES

DM is characterized by chronic hyperglycemia resulting from defects in insulin secretion, insulin action, or both.[6] There are several pathophysiologic processes that occur leading to the development of type 2 DM (T2DM). These processes are described as follows.

Beta-Cell Failure

The β-cells of the pancreas are no longer producing enough insulin to match physiologic needs, leading to greater amounts of circulating glucose and hyperglycemia.

Insulin Resistance

Insulin may have a reduced effect, leading to lessened peripheral glucose uptake and higher blood glucose (BG).

Inappropriate Hormone Release

In T2DM, the feedback systems for hepatic glucose production and glucagon release are defective, leading to inappropriate glucose release from the liver and glucagon release from the alpha cells of the pancreas, even when sugars are normal or high.

Decreased Incretin Effect

The incretin hormones of the intestines aid in food digestion and promoting feelings of satiety. The 2 main incretin hormones, GIP and GLP-1, are instrumental in promoting insulin release and inhibiting glucagon production. Individuals with T2DM have a poor response to incretin hormones, leading to poor carbohydrate absorption and delivery and hyperglycemia.

The development of T2DM is a heterogenous condition involving multiple factors including genetics and environment.[7] T1DM is an autoimmune process in which the islet cells of the pancreas are attacked by the body, leading to no insulin production. Similar to T2DM, there are many factors likely involved in the development of T1DM including genetic susceptibility, ineffective immune response, and inflammation.[6]

DIAGNOSIS OF TYPE 1 DIABETES VERSUS TYPE 2 DIABETES

Although there are at least 5 classifications of diabetes including prediabetes, T1DM and T2DM are the 2 predominant types. Evidence affirms that T2DM accounts for approximately 90% to 95% of diabetes cases.[8] The symptoms of T1DM and T2DM are similar; however, there are key clinical findings (**Table 1**) that are specific to each type that are helpful in guiding a correct diagnosis. These defining characteristics are necessary to properly guide assessment, diagnosis, planning, interventions, evaluations, treatment regimens, and research efforts.

MANAGEMENT OF TYPE 1 DIABETES VERSUS TYPE 2 DIABETES

Although diagnostic criteria are similar for both T1DM and T2DM, the treatment approach is considerably different. Patients with T1DM require exogenous insulin throughout their lifetimes due to the autoimmune destruction of the beta cells, leaving the body deficient of endogenous insulin. Subsequently, administration of basal and bolus insulin via multiple injections or insulin pump devices is necessary to sustain life in patients with T1DM.

For people with T2DM, metformin, along with diet and lifestyle changes, is typically initiated as first-line therapy. Developments of new pharmacologic agents often pose

Table 1
Comparison and characteristics of type 1 diabetes and type 2 diabetes

Feature	Type 1 Diabetes	Type 2 Diabetes
Diagnostic criteria	• HBA1C >6.5 or FPG ≥126 mg/dL (7.0 mmol/L)[a] • Oral glucose tolerance test 2-hour plasma glucose ≥200 mg/dL[a] • Hyperglycemia symptoms and random plasma glucose ≥200	
Autoantibodies	Positive glutamic acid decarboxylase	Negative
Etiology	Genetic, environmental, and autoimmune factors, idiopathic	Genetic, obesity (central adipose), sedentary lifestyle, GDM, metabolic syndrome
Onset	Sudden (wk), often present acutely with ketoacidosis	Gradual (mo to y)
Age	Any age	Any age (primarily adults)
Body habitus	Thin or normal	Obese, often central abdominal obesity
Symptoms at onset	Extremely high blood sugars, weight loss, frequent urination, diabetes ketoacidosis, yeast infection	High blood sugars, fatigue, increased thirst, increased hunger, increased urination
Treatment	Exogenous insulin	Diet, exercise, oral hypoglycemic agents, exogenous insulin
Endogenous insulin (C-peptide)	Low or absent	Normal, decreased
Insulin resistance	Not present	Present

Abbreviation: GDM, gestational diabetes mellitus.
[a] Results should generally be confirmed by repeat testing.
Data from Kharroubi AT, Darwish HM. Diabetes mellitus: the epidemic of the century. World J Diabetes 2015;6(6):850–67.

a challenge for clinicians with the ever-increasing classes and combinations of medications, making diabetes one of the most complex chronic illnesses to treat in primary care. Fortunately, expert panels have carefully developed clinical guideline algorithms that can easily translate clinical practice to assist patients in achieving glycemic control. A review of available medications to treat diabetes is listed in **Table 2**. All patients with T2DM should implement lifestyle and nonpharmacologic modifications, such as a low-calorie, low-carbohydrate diet, and at least 150 minutes per week of moderate-intensity exercise to optimize quality of life, reduce complications, and improve glycemic control.[8]

GOALS OF DIABETES TREATMENT

Because cardiovascular disease (CVD) is the primary cause of death in people with diabetes, the overarching goal of diabetes management is cardiovascular risk reduction (CRR). CRR is achieved through optimal BG levels, blood pressure management, statin therapy, tobacco cessation, weight reduction, a healthy diet, and physical activity.[8] An overview of recommendations for CRR is listed in **Table 3**.

Clinical practice guidelines exist to offer integrated treatment approaches that involve both the patient and the primary care provider in selecting the best treatment options to achieve goals. Abundant research has confirmed that elevated blood

Table 2
Current medications available to treat diabetes mellitus

Medication Class		Route	Average HbA1c Reduction	Potential for Hypoglycemia	Impact on Weight	Cost	Contraindications	Side Effects
Insulin	Insulin (prandial) Short-acting Regular Rapid-acting analog Lispro Aspart Glulisine	Injection	1.0%–1.5%	Moderate-high	↑ Weight	Inexpensive (human insulin) Moderate to expensive (analogs)	• Hypersensitivity • Hypoglycemia	• Hypoglycemia • Injection site reaction • Lipodystrophy
	Insulin (basal) Intermediate acting NPH Long-acting analogs Glargine Detemir Degludec	Injection	1.0%–1.5%	Moderate-high	↑ Weight	Inexpensive (human insulin) Moderate to expensive (analogs)	• IV administration • Hypersensitivity • Hypoglycemia	• Hypoglycemia • Injection site reaction • Lipodystrophy
	Premixed NPH/Regular Biphasic insulin aspart Insulin Lispro Protamine/Lispro Insulin Degludec/aspart	Injection	1.0%–1.5%	Moderate-high	↑ Weight	Inexpensive (human insulin) Moderate to expensive (analogs)	• Hypersensitivity • Hypoglycemia	• Hypoglycemia • Injection site reaction • Lipodystrophy
Biguanide	Metformin	Oral	1.0%–1.5%	Low	Weight neutral	Inexpensive	• Hypersensitivity • eGFR <46 • Metabolic acidosis • Diabetic ketoacidosis (DKA) • Lactic acidosis	• GI Symptoms (diarrhea, n/v, flatulence)

Class	Drugs	Route		Effect	Cost	Contraindications	Side Effects
Sulfonylurea	Glipizide Glyburide Chlorpropamide Tolazamide Tolbutamide	Oral	1.0%–1.5%	Moderate	↑ Weight	Inexpensive	• Hypersensitivity • DKA • Near-term pregnancy	• Hypoglycemia • Nausea/Vomiting • Anorexia
Thiazolidines	Pioglitazone Rosiglitazone	Oral	1.0%–1.5%	Low	↑ Weight	Inexpensive (pioglitazone) Moderately expensive (rosiglitazone)	• T1DM • DKA • Active bladder ca • CHF, NYHA, Class III–IV • Baseline • Pediatric patients • Symptomatic CHF	• URI • H/A • Myalgia • Weight gain • Flatulence
GLP-1 agonists	Lixisenatide Exenatide Albiglutide Liraglutide Lixisenatide Dulaglutide	Injection	1.0–1.5%	Low	↓Weight	Expensive	• T1DM • Pancreatitis Hx • DKA • Gastroparesis, severe • Hypersensitivity • IM or IV administration • Weigh risk vs benefit in pregnancy • -Consider alternative if breastfeeding	• N/V • H/A • Diarrhea • Dizziness • Injection site reaction • Abdomen pain

(continued on next page)

Table 2
(continued)

Medication Class	Route	Average HbA1c Reduction	Potential for Hypoglycemia	Impact on Weight	Cost	Contraindications	Side Effects
DPP-IV inhibitors Sitagliptin Alogliptin Saxagliptin Linagliptin	Oral	0.5%–1.0%	Low	Weight neutral	Expensive	• T1DM • DKA • Pancreatitis Hx • Crcl <50 • Caution in pregnancy • Consider alternative if breastfeeding	• URI • H/A • Diarrhea • Abdominal pain
Meglitinides Nateglinide Repaglinide		0.5%–1.0%	Moderate	↑ Weight	Inexpensive (repaglinide) Moderately expensive (nateglinide)	• Hypersensitivity • T1DM • DKA • Caution in pregnancy • Consider alternative if breastfeeding	• Hypoglycemia • Headache • Arthralgia • UTI
Amylin analog Pramlintide	Injection	0.5%–1.0%	High	↓Weight	Expensive	• Hypersensitivity • Pediatric Patients • Hypoglycemia unawareness • HbA1c >9% • Gastroparesis • Caution in pregnancy • Consider alternative if breastfeeding	• Nausea/Vomiting • Headache • Anorexia • Abdominal pain

Class	Generic	Route	A1c	Hypoglycemia	Weight	Cost	Contraindications/Cautions	Side effects
Alpha glucose inhibitors	Acarbose Miglitol	Oral	0.5%–1.0%	Low	Weight Neutral	Inexpensive (acarbose) Moderately expensive (miglitol)	• Hypersensitivity • DKA • Cirrhosis • Colonic ulcer • Partial GI obstruction • Cr >2.0 • Caution in pregnancy • Consider alternative if breastfeeding	• Flatulence • Diarrhea • Abdominal pain • Elevated LFTs
Sodium-glucose co-transporter 2 inhibitors (SGLT-2)	Canagliflozin Dapagliflozin Empagliflozin	Oral	0.5%–1.0%	Low	↓Weight	Expensive	• Hypersensitivity • Pregnancy 2nd or 3rd trimester • T1DM • DKA • Volume depletion • eGFR <45 • Caution in pregnancy • Consider alternative if breastfeeding	• Hyperkalemia • Hypoglycemia • UTI

Abbreviations: ↑, higher or gain; ↓, lower or loss; ca, cancer; CHF, congestive heart failure; CrCl, creatinine clearance; DKA, diabetic ketoacidosis; DPP-IV inhibitors, dipeptidyl peptidase 4 inhibitors; eGFR, estimated glomerular filtration rate; GI, gastrointestinal; H/A, headache; Hx, history; IM, intramuscular; IV, intravenous; LFT, liver function tests; n/v or N/V, nausea and vomiting; NPH, neutral protamine hagedorn; NYHA, New York Heart Association; T1DM, type 1 diabetes mellitus; URI, upper respiratory infection; UTI, urinary tract infection.

Adapted from Department of Veterans Affairs, Department of Defense. VA/DoD clinical practice guideline for the management of type 2 diabetes mellitus in primary care. 2017. Available at: https://www.healthquality.va.gov/guidelines/cd/diabetes/. Accessed June 26, 2017.

Table 3
Clinical guidelines for cardiovascular risk reduction in diabetes

Clinical Guidelines for Cardiovascular Risk Reduction in Diabetes (American Diabetes Association, 2017)	
Blood glucose targets	A1c 7% or less for most A1c 6.5% may be appropriate for some younger, healthier patients (if achieved without hypoglycemia) Avoiding hypoglycemia
Blood pressure targets	140/90 130/80: May be appropriate for some younger patients, if it can be achieved without harm
Cholesterol	Moderate to high-intensity statin
Diet/lifestyle	Weight reduction (start with 5% of body weight) 150 min of moderate activity/wk; Combination of aerobic and weight training Tobacco cessation Alcohol: 1 drink/d (women); 2 drinks/d (men) (1 ounce of liquor, 4 ounces wine, 12 ounces beer)

Data from Marathe PH, Gao HX, Close KL. American Diabetes Association standards of medical care in diabetes 2017. J Diabetes 2017;9(4):320–4.

glucose and HbA1c values over time are directly correlated to the development of both microvascular and macrovascular complications.[9] Interestingly, 33% to 49% of patients do not meet glycemic, blood pressure, or cholesterol target goals; major factors that contribute to developing microvascular and macrovascular complications.[8]

Traditionally, health care providers aimed for all patients with diabetes to keep their HbA1c values below 7% (8.5 mmol/L) to reduce microvascular complications. However, adaptation to recent changes in clinical guidelines implemented by the American Association of Clinical Endocrinologists and the American Diabetes Association suggest tailoring HbA1c values according to patients' life expectancy, disease duration, hypoglycemia risk, established vascular complications, presence of relevant comorbidities, and social determinants of health.[8] Thus, the HbA1c target for patients with long life expectancy, short duration of diabetes, and low risk of hypoglycemia without CVD is 6.5% (7.8 mmol/L). An HbA1c less than 8% (10.1 mmol/L) is acceptable for patients with history of severe hypoglycemia, limited life expectancy, advanced microvascular or macrovascular complications, extensive comorbid conditions, and long-standing diabetes.[10]

Self-management approaches are essential and effective to improve glycemic control and decrease the risk of complications. Additional recommended self-management behaviors include frequent blood glucose monitoring, medication adherence, following nutritional health plans that limit high fat and carbohydrate foods, and smoking cessation. Additionally, diabetes self-management education (DSME) programs are also available to assist patients who need additional encouragement and education necessary to improve self-management practices and reach optimal glycemic targets. Overall, a significant improvement in HbA1c values resulting in a reduction of cardiovascular complications is achieved when collaborative, integrated efforts exist among patients, health care providers, and DSME members.[11] Other preventive practices to reduce diabetes complications include annual dilated eye examinations, annual foot examinations, self-management education classes, and daily blood glucose monitoring.

COMPLICATIONS OF DIABETES: MICROVASCULAR AND MACROVASCULAR DISEASE

Cardiovascular events are the most prevalent cause of morbidity and mortality in patients with diabetes.[12] Patients with diabetes and hyperglycemia often develop hypertension and dyslipidemia and this deadly triad increases the risk of developing macrovascular complications. Uncontrolled diabetes is the largest contributor to heart disease and stroke in the United States and is the primary source of chronic kidney disease worldwide.[9] Diabetes is the main culprit responsible for 50% of nontraumatic foot amputations.[13] More information about the prevalence of common diabetes complications is listed in **Table 4**.

COMPLICATIONS OF DIABETES: DIABETIC KETOACIDOSIS AND HYPERGLYCEMIC HYPEROSMOLAR STATE
Epidemiology

Diabetic ketoacidosis (DKA) and hyperglycemic hyperosmolar state (HHS) represent 2 of the most common, life-threatening complications of DM[14] that can rapidly lead to organ failure if not treated quickly. These endocrine hyperglycemic emergencies are associated with morbidity and mortality, reduced life expectancy, and significant health care costs.[15] In the United States, hospital admission rates for DKA increased by 30% over the past decade.[16] Approximately 145,000 cases of DKA occur each year in the United States.[17] DKA inpatient mortality in the United States is less than 1%.

Table 4
Common microvascular and macrovascular complications in patients with diabetes

Complications		Type 1 Diabetes	Type 2 Diabetes
Macrovascular complications	Coronary artery disease	Adults with diabetes are 2–4 times more likely to die from heart disease than adults without diabetes	
	Peripheral artery disease		Estimated 14% of patients with T2DM have PAD
	Stroke	People with diabetes have double the risk of an ischemic stroke compared with general population	
		Estimated 7%–12% of patients with diabetes will have an ischemic stroke	
		Risk of stroke increases 3% each y of diabetes and risk triples after 10 y of diabetes	
Microvascular complications	Nephropathy	25%–50% risk for developing chronic kidney disease	Occurs in approximately 38% Will most likely progress to ESRD than patients with T1DM
	Neuropathy	Up to 32% of patients with T1DM will develop peripheral neuropathy	Up to 48% of patients with T2DM may develop peripheral neuropathy
	Retinopathy	PDR is the most common vision-threatening lesion particularly among patients with T1DM	Approximately 33% of patients with diabetes have signs of diabetic retinopathy

Abbreviations: ESRD, end-stage renal disease; PAD, peripheral arterial disease; PDR, proliferative diabetic retinopathy; T1DM, type 1 diabetes mellitus; T2DM, type 2 diabetes mellitus.
Data from Refs.[12,23–29]

HHS is less common, and hospital admission rates account for less than 1% of all diabetes-related admissions.[16] However, HHS inpatient mortality is higher than DKA, ranging from 5% to 16%.[17] Hyperglycemic emergencies are estimated to cost US hospitals $2.4 billion[16] per year, averaging $17,500 per patient.[17] With the growing prevalence of diabetes in the United States, treatment costs for these life-threatening complications will likely continue to grow.

DKA is predominately seen in T1DM, but can occur in patients with T2DM who are obese and without autoimmune markers. Female patients, children younger than 18 years, ethnic minorities, those with hemoglobin A1c of 7.5% or greater, and those with a longer duration of diabetes have the highest risk factors for DKA.[18]

The exact incidence of HHS is unknown. HHS is predominately seen in patients older than 60 years with T2DM.[19] HHS is seen more often in those previously diagnosed with diabetes than in those newly diagnosed,[17] and among individuals of African American ethnicity.[20]

Pathophysiology

DKA and HHS both result from an absolute or relative insulin deficiency with a subsequent increase in counter-regulatory hormones, such as glucagon, catecholamines, cortisol, and growth hormone.[16] Any residual insulin is opposed once this hormonal cascade begins leading to increased hepatic glucose production, decreased peripheral insulin sensitivity, hyperglycemia, and dehydration and electrolyte abnormalities resulting from osmotic diuresis caused by glycosuria.[17] Although similar in pathophysiology, DKA and HHS differ in the degree of metabolic acidosis, ketosis, and dehydration.[17]

DKA consists of the triad of hyperglycemia, hyperketonemia, and metabolic acidosis secondary to the deterioration of fatty acid metabolism.[21] Free fatty acids (FFAs) are released from adipose tissue into circulation (lipolysis) in response to relative or absolute insulin deficiency. FFAs are oxidized in the liver to ketone bodies (acetoacetate and B-hydroxybutyrate) resulting in hyperketonemia. Excess ketones spill over into the urine causing ketonuria. Increased production of ketone bodies eventually leads to decreased bicarbonate and metabolic acidosis.[16]

HHS consists of severe hyperglycemia, hyperosmolality, and dehydration without significant ketosis.[19] Glucose and counter-regulatory hormones increase the vascular space. To maintain homeostasis, an osmotic fluid shift from the intravascular space to the vascular space begins.[17] At the same time, osmotic diuresis occurs, causing electrolyte imbalances, mainly with sodium and potassium. Acidosis does not occur with HHS, possibly due to a sufficient amount of insulin available to inhibit the breakdown of FFA for fuel.[17]

DKA is associated with abnormality of blood coagulation and increased risk of thrombosis formation, predisposing the individual to potentially fatal complications that include stroke, myocardial infarction, and disseminated intravascular coagulation.[18] Acute respiratory failure and acute renal failure due to severe dehydration and coma are other potentially fatal complications. Reasons for death in DKA/HHS are mainly attributed to the precipitating cause, advanced age, and severity of dehydration.[16]

Diagnosis

In a hyperglycemic emergency, a prompt yet accurate diagnosis is needed to determine the appropriate course of treatment. DKA and HHS should be considered in all ill patients presenting with hyperglycemia.[17] There are similarities and notable differences in the presenting signs and symptoms, physical examination, and laboratory findings between DKA and HHS. The primary precipitating factor for DKA and HHS is infection.[16] Infection is the most common cause of DKA in T1DM, followed by inadequate use of insulin, insulin omission, or discontinuation of insulin (17-Umpierrez). Delay in seeking medical care for an infection (urinary tract infection, pneumonia) in the elderly is the most common cause of HHS.[16] Other precipitating factors for development of DKA and HHS include cardiovascular events, pancreatitis, alcohol use, cocaine use, depression, eating disorders, insulin pump failure, noncompliance with antidiabetic regimen, and certain medications (such as glucocorticoids, antipsychotics, beta-blockers, sodium-glucose co-transporter 2 inhibitors, thiazide diuretics).[16,22] Refer to Kitabchi and colleagues[15] for a comprehensive table denoting the diagnostic criteria for DKA.

Presenting Signs and Symptoms

In DKA, presenting signs and symptoms are typically acute onset. Patients commonly report symptoms including polydipsia, polyuria, sudden weight loss (newly diagnosed T1DM), nausea, vomiting, and abdominal pain. Approximately half of patients will report abdominal pain and up to two-thirds of patients will report nausea and vomiting.[16] Lethargy and stupor are seen in half of patients presenting with DKA and approximately 25% present with loss of consciousness.[16]

In HHS, presenting signs and symptoms may develop over a period of days to weeks. Symptoms commonly include polydipsia, polyuria, weakness, blurred vision, weight loss, and mental status decline.[16,17,20]

Physical Examination Findings

In DKA, poor skin turgor, tachycardia, dehydration with dry mucous membranes, hypotension, and Kussmaul (deep, labored breathing) respirations and fruity (acetone) breath odor (resulting from the metabolic acidosis) may be present. Examination findings for HHS are similar to DKA and include significant signs of dehydration.[20]

Laboratory Findings

DKA and HHS are diagnosed based on laboratory evaluation of plasma glucose, arterial pH, serum bicarbonate, urine and serum ketones, effective serum osmolality and anion gap, and mental status. If concurrent illness is suspected, appropriate additional laboratory and diagnostics should be considered.

Plasma glucose values for DKA are usually greater than 250 mg/dL. It is important to note that not all patients with DKA may have hyperglycemia. Euglycemic DKA is seen in approximately 10% of those who develop DKA and demonstrate a glucose level less than or equal to 250 mg/dL.[16] DKA is classified as mild, moderate, or severe depending on the degree of acidosis. Most patients present with mild to moderate DKA. Elevation in serum concentration of ketone bodies is the key diagnostic criteria for DKA.[17] Ketone body production is typically measured by direct measurement of *B*-hydroxybutyrate, the ketone body that is produced most prevalently in DKA.[20]

Once therapy is initiated, capillary glucose should be checked every 1 to 2 hours and serum electrolytes, blood glucose, urea nitrogen, creatinine, and venous pH every 4 hours. Cardiac monitoring for irregular rhythms before, during, and after therapy should also be initiated.

TREATMENT

Medical management of DKA and HHS requires intravenous (IV) replacement of fluid and electrolytes to correct the dehydration, administration of insulin to correct the hyperglycemia, and treatment for any underlying cause if one is present. Correction of the fluid deficit with IV fluids is a critical first step to restore renal perfusion and intravascular volume. Circulating counter-regulator hormones are decreased when intravascular volume is restored, resulting in decreased insulin resistance. In HHS, when proper fluid resuscitation is provided, patients may see an improvement in mental status.

Intravenous Fluids

The expected fluid deficit in DKA can range from 3 to 5 L, and in HHS can be >9 L.[16] The preferred solution for fluid resuscitation is isotonic saline (0.9% NaCl). For the first 2 to 4 hours, normal saline is administered at a rate of 500 to 1000 mL/h. After correction of volume depletion has been accomplished, the infusion rate of normal saline is reduced to 250 mL/h or switched to 0.45% saline (250–500 mL/h) depending on serum sodium levels. Replacement fluids should change to 5% dextrose when plasma blood glucose reaches 200 mg/L to avoid hypoglycemia and allow for ongoing concomitant administration of insulin to correct ketonemia.[15,17]

Insulin Therapy

Regular human insulin administered intravenously is the treatment of choice. Many clinicians begin with an IV bolus of 0.1 U/kg, followed by a continuous insulin infusion of 0.1 U/kg per hour. The insulin rate should be reduced to 0.05 U/kg per hour when glucose levels are ≤250 mg/dL. From that point, the rate should be adjusted to maintain a glucose level of 200 mg/dL. For patients with mild DKA, subcutaneous rapid-acting insulin analogs are an alternative option to IV insulin.[15]

Potassium

Initiation of insulin therapy should commence only when serum potassium levels are greater than 3.3 mEq/L. This is important because insulin therapy promotes movement of potassium back into the intracellular compartment. If insulin therapy is initiated when potassium levels are now, life-threatening hypokalemia may occur. **Table 5** includes guidelines for potassium replacement.

Bicarbonate

Use of bicarbonate is not routinely recommended in DKA and is not administered in HHS. Consider administration of 50 to 100 mmol/L in 500 mL of 0.45% saline if pH

Table 5
Potassium replacement guidelines

Serum K + Level, mEq/L	Potassium Replacement
>5	No replacement needed
4–5	Add 20 mEq/L potassium chloride to IVF
3–4	Add 40 mEq/L potassium chloride to IVF
<3	10–20 mEq/*hour* added to IVF • Once K is >3 mEq; add 40 mEq/L to IVF • Hold insulin until K is >3.3 mEq

Abbreviation: IVF, intravenous fluids.

Data from Fayman M, Pasquel FJ, Umpierrez GE. Management of hyperglycemic crisis diabetic ketoacidosis and hyperglycemic hyperosmolar state. Med Clin N Am 2017;101:587–606; and Tran TT, Pease A, Wood AJ, et al. Review of evidence for adult diabetic ketoacidosis management protocols. Front Endocrinol 2017;8:106.

is <6.9. This is run over 1 hour and until the pH increases to greater than or equal to 7.0. Bicarbonate is not administered if pH is greater than or equal to 7.0.[17]

Phosphate

Use of phosphate is not routinely required for patients with DKA. Once a patient resumes eating, the mild hypophosphatemia seen in DKA generally corrects itself. Consideration for phosphate repletion is reserved for patients with respiratory or cardiac distress with serum phosphate levels less than 0.32 mmol/L.[17]

Maintenance Therapy

The resolution criteria for DKA include a plasma glucose level less than 250 mg/dL, serum bicarbonate level ≥18 mmol/L, normalization of the anion gap, and arterial pH >7.3. The resolution criteria for HHS is defined as an effective serum osmolality <310 mmol/kg and plasma glucose level ≤250 mg/dL in a mentally alert patient.[15,17]

Switching to subcutaneous insulin is considered when the resolution criteria for DKA and HHS are met and the patient is alert and able to eat food. Insulin therapy should continue for 2 to 4 hours after subcutaneous insulin is started to prevent rebound hyperglycemia and recurrent ketoacidosis.[16] Those previously using subcutaneous insulin before hospitalization can resume their prior regimen. Basal/bolus regimens with insulin analogs are preferred over intermediate insulin and regular insulin for newly diagnosed patients.[17]

Patient-centered diabetes education is critical to avoiding hyperglycemic emergencies. Patients should be equipped to handle sick days and understand the signs and symptoms to be aware of should infection or illness occur.

SUMMARY

DM and its complications are among the leading causes of organ failure around the world. It is imperative that timely, patient-centered care is provided to avoid microvascular and macrovascular damage. People with well-controlled diabetes can live long and healthy lives through interprofessional management, emphasizing optimal, individualized care.

REFERENCES

1. Weng J, Hu G. Diabetes: leveraging the tipping point of the diabetes pandemic. Diabetes 2017;66(6):1461–3.
2. Forouhi NG, Wareham NJ. Epidemiology of diabetes. Medicine 2014;42(12):698–702.
3. United States, Centers for Disease Control and Prevention. National Diabetes Statistics Report, 2014 Fast Facts - Data and Statistics About Diabetes. 2017. Available at: https://www.cdc.gov/nchs/fastats/diabetes.htm. Accessed June 22, 2017.
4. Chaudhury A, Duvoor C, Dendi VS, et al. Clinical review of antidiabetic drugs: implications for type 2 diabetes mellitus management. Front Endocrinol 2017;8:1–12.
5. United States, Centers for disease control and prevention, National Center for Health Statistics. Deaths and Mortality, 2017. Available at: https://www.cdc.gov/nchs/fastats/deaths.htm. Accessed June 22, 2017.
6. Ozougwu JC, Obimba KC, Belonwu CD, et al. The pathogenesis and pathophysiology of type 1 and type 2 diabetes mellitus. J Physiol Pathophysiology 2013;4(4):46–57.

7. Kahn SE, Cooper ME, Prato SD. Pathophysiology and treatment of type 2 diabetes: perspectives on the past, present, and future. Lancet 2014;383.9922: 1068–83.

8. American Diabetes Association. Standards of medical care in diabetes, 2017. Diabetes Care 2017;40(1):1–142.

9. Phillips LS, Ratner RE, Buse JB, et al. We can change the natural history of type 2 diabetes. Diabetes Care 2014;37(10):2668–76.

10. Brateanu A, Russo-Alvarez G, Nielsen C. Starting insulin in patients with type 2 diabetes: an individualized approach. Cleve Clin J Med 2015;82(8):513–9.

11. Chrvala CA, Sherr D, Lipman RD. Diabetes self-management education for adults with type 2 diabetes mellitus: a systematic review of the effect on glycemic control. Patient Education Couns 2016;99(6):926–43.

12. Leon BM, Maddox TM. Diabetes and cardiovascular disease: epidemiology, biological mechanisms, treatment recommendations and future research. World J Diabetes 2015;6(13):1246–58.

13. Jha V, Garcia-Garcia G, Iseki K, et al. Chronic kidney disease: global dimension and perspectives. Lancet 2013;382(9888):260–72.

14. Bradford AL, Crider CC, Xu X, et al. Predictors of recurrent hospital admission for patients presenting with diabetic ketoacidosis and hyperglycemic hyperosmolar state. J Clin Med Res 2017;9(1):35–9.

15. Kitabchi AE, Miles JM, Umpierrez GE, et al. American Diabetes Association consensus statement hyperglycemic crisis in adult patients with diabetes. Diabetes Care 2009;32:1335–43.

16. Fayman M, Pasquel FJ, Umpierrez GE. Management of hyperglycemic crisis diabetic ketoacidosis and hyperglycemic hyperosmolar state. Med Clin North Am 2017;101:587–606.

17. Umipierrez G, Korytkowski M. Diabetic emergencies–ketoacidosis, hyperglycaemic hyperosmolar state and hypoglycaemia. Nat Rev Endocrinol 2016;12: 222–32.

18. Tran TT, Pease A, Wood AJ, et al. Review of evidence for adult diabetic ketoacidosis management protocols. Front Endocrinol 2017;8:106.

19. Pasqeul FJ, Umipierrez GE. Hyperosmolar hyperglycemic state: a historic review of the clinical presentation, diagnosis and treatment. Diabetes Care 2014;37: 3124–31.

20. McCombs DG, Appel SJ, Ward ME. Expedited diagnosis and management of inpatient hyperosmolar hyperglycemia nonketotic syndrome. J Am Assoc Nurse Pract 2015;27:426–32.

21. Kamata Y, Takano K, Kishihara E, et al. Distinct clinical characteristics and therapeutic modalities for diabetic ketoacidosis in type 1 and type 2 diabetes mellitus. J Diabetes Complications 2017;31:468–72.

22. Echouffo-Tcheugue J, Garg R. Management of hyperglycemia and diabetes in the emergency department. Curr Diab Rep 2017;17:56.

23. Ou H, Yang C, Wang J, et al. Life expectancy and lifetime health care expenditures for type 1 diabetes: a nationwide longitudinal cohort of incident cases followed for 14 years. Value Health 2016;19(8):976–84.

24. United States Renal Data System. 2016 USRDS annual data report: epidemiology of kidney disease in the United States. Bethesda (MD): National Institutes of Health, National Institute of Diabetes and Digestive and Kidney Diseases; 2016.

25. Criqui MH, Aboyans V. Epidemiology of peripheral artery disease. Circ Res 2015; 116(9):1509–26.

26. Banerjee C, Moon YP, Paik MC, et al. Duration of diabetes and risk of ischemic stroke. Stroke 2012;43(5):1212–7.
27. Luitse MJ, Biessels GJ, Rutten GE, et al. Diabetes, hyperglycaemia, and acute ischaemic stroke. Lancet Neurol 2012;11(3):261–71.
28. Nathan DM, DCCT/Edic Research Group. The diabetes control and complications trial/epidemiology of diabetes interventions and complications study at 30 years: overview. Diabetes care 2014;37(1):9–16.
29. Ismail-Beigi F, Craven T, Banerji MA, et al. Effect of intensive treatment of hyperglycaemia on microvascular outcomes in type 2 diabetes: an analysis of the ACCORD randomised trial. Lancet 2010;376(9739):419–30.

Immunosuppressive/ Autoimmune Disorders

Angela Richard-Eaglin, DNP, MSN, APRN, FNP-BC[a],*,
Benjamin A. Smallheer, PhD, RN, ACNP-BC, FNP-BC, CCRN, CNE[b]

KEYWORDS

- Autoimmune disorders • Graves disease • Hashimoto thyroiditis
- Inflammatory bowel disease • Crohn disease • Ulcerative colitis
- Systemic lupus erythematosus • Multiple sclerosis

KEY POINTS

- There are nearly 100 autoimmune diseases and the most prevalent are type 1 diabetes and autoimmune thyroid disease.
- Autoimmune thyroid disease is the most common autoimmune disorder.
- Clinical presentation and clinical management of autoimmune disorders are based on the disease type.

BACKGROUND

Autoimmune disorders refer to a category of diseases in which the immune system attacks healthy cells in the body.[1] Evidence suggests that exposure to antigens from bacteria, viruses, toxins, and blood and tissue from external sources trigger an immune response in which the body mistakenly attacks healthy cells in an attempt to rid itself of harmful substances.[1,2] As a result, the following adverse events may occur: tissue damage, malfunctions in organ growth, and organ dysfunction.[1]

Following cancer and heart disease, autoimmune diseases are the third most common disease category, affecting approximately 8% of the population.[1] Women are affected at an approximately 75% higher rate than men, and the disease onset often occurs during the childbearing years, from the ages of 14 to 44 years.[2–5] Autoimmune diseases can affect almost every body system, including neurologic, cardiac, endocrine, musculoskeletal, gastrointestinal (GI), lung, kidney, skin, eye, and vascular

Disclosure: The authors do not have any relationship with a commercial company that has a direct financial interest in subject matter or materials discussed in article or with a company making a competing product.
[a] Healthcare in Adult Populations Division, Duke University School of Nursing, DUMC 3322, 307 Trent Drive, Durham, NC 27710, USA; [b] Adult-Gerontology Acute Care Nurse Practitioner Program, Duke University School of Nursing, 307 Trent Drive, Durham, NC 27710, USA
* Corresponding author.
E-mail address: angela.richard-eaglin@duke.edu

https://doi.org/10.1016/j.cnur.2018.04.002
0029-6465/18/© 2018 Elsevier Inc. All rights reserved.
nursing.theclinics.com

systems.[6] Some autoimmune disorders are organ specific, whereas a host of immunologic dysfunctions lead to involvement of multiple organs.[5] Over the last decade, substantial improvements have been made in the diagnosis and classification of autoimmune diseases, which have brought improvements in prognosis.[5] Diagnosis, prognosis, epidemiology, treatment, and complications are disease specific, and are discussed here by disease type.

CAUSE

Autoimmune diseases are caused by a dysfunction of the acquired immune system. These diseases can affect any system in the body and are initiated when the immune system becomes overactive and, rather than destroying invader cells, targets the body's own healthy cells and tissues.[3] Unlike the innate immune system, which is present at birth and does not use antibodies for activation, the antibodies and immune cells of the acquired immune system inappropriately target the body's own healthy tissues, signaling immune cells to attack and destroy them.[6] There is no definitive cause of autoimmune disorders.[1,6,7] However, autoimmune responses have been found to be linked to a genetic predisposition that increases the likelihood of disease development when exposed to environmental triggers.[1,5–7] In most cases, a combination of genetic predisposition, organic influences such as stress and hormonal activity, and environmental factors influence development of autoimmune disease.[1,3,5–7] Examples of these environmental factors that contribute to autoimmune disorder development include infections (bacterial, viral, or parasitic) and various environmental influences, such as medications and toxic chemicals, dietary components, occupational exposures, smoking, and decreases in vitamin D levels.[5,6,8,9]

The concept of immune tolerance also suggests that the immune system typically has the ability to prevent itself from targeting self-molecules, tissues, or cells. Within the thymus, developing lymphocytes undergo a complex process of differentiation and programming of self versus nonself, known as positive selection. Lymphocytes with potential reactivity against self-peptides are negatively selected and therefore destroyed by the body. Once these mature T cells exit the thymus, they are subjected to peripheral selection and further screened by the body for self-reactivity and again may be deleted.[5,10] It is suggested that this process of positive and negative selection may be an initial key factor in the development of autoimmune disorders.

COMMON TYPES OF AUTOIMMUNE DISORDERS

There are nearly 100 autoimmune diseases, and the 2 most prevalent types are type 1 diabetes mellitus (T1DM) and autoimmune thyroid disease (AITD).[5] However, T1DM is not discussed in this article. Graves disease (GD) and Hashimoto thyroiditis (HT) are the main AITDs.[11,12] In addition, other commonly diagnosed autoimmune disorders are rheumatoid arthritis (RA), inflammatory bowel disease (IBD; Crohn disease and ulcerative colitis), systemic lupus erythematosus (SLE), and multiple sclerosis (MS).[1,5–7]

Autoimmune Thyroid Disorders

The most common and the most frequently occurring autoimmune disorder is AITD, which is T-cell mediated and organ specific.[11] AITD affects about 5% of the population and is more common in women than in men.[11] There is evidence to support genetic susceptibility to AITD, but certain environmental factors, such as infection, stress, smoking cigarettes, medications, radiation, and iodine, also contribute to the development of AITD.[11–14] AITD occurs when the immune system becomes dysregulated and causes an attack on the thyroid.[14] The 2 main types of AITD are GD and HT, both of which are characterized by infiltration of lymphocytes to the parenchyma of the thyroid.[14] GD may evolve into HT and vice versa, which is an indication that the two disorders possess pathophysiologic similarities.[15]

HT is defined as chronic thyroid gland inflammation and is also known as chronic lymphocytic thyroiditis.[13–15] It is the most common autoimmune disease and often leads to hypothyroidism.[11–15] It is frequently associated with T1DM.[11] HT is classified as either primary or secondary, based on presence or lack of an cause.[13] Cases of HT with no identifiable cause are classified as primary, and this is the most common form of thyroiditis.[13] Secondary HT includes forms of HT with a definitive, identifiable cause, and is most commonly induced by immunomodulatory drugs.[13] HT can occur at any age but is most prevalent in middle-aged women; however, it can also occur in men and in children.[14] It affects white and Asian people more than African Americans.[13]

Although not observed in all patients with GD, it is often characterized by a triad of disorders, which include thyrotoxicosis, ophthalmopathy, and goiter.[12,16] Often, the only clinical feature in patients with GD is hyperthyroidism.[12] The exact cause of GD is unknown; however, individuals with GD exhibit loss of immune tolerance to thyroid antigens, which triggers the body's attack on the thyroid.[12] Specifically, circulating antibodies mimic the action of thyroid-stimulating hormone (TSH), which creates an increase in the synthesis and release of thyroid hormones, thus causing hyperthyroidism and thyroid hypertrophy (goiter).[12] About 50% of patients develop ophthalmopathy, which is the most common extrathyroidal feature of GD.[12]

Rheumatoid Arthritis

RA is a chronic inflammatory disease that occurs when the body attacks the joints, resulting in chronic systemic inflammation, synovitis, and pain.[6,17–19] The chronic inflammation associated with RA may be debilitating, secondary to bone and cartilage damage.[19] RA primarily manifests in the joints, but it also involves rheumatoid nodules, the pulmonary system, and often causes systemic comorbidities.[6,17–19] It affects approximately 1% of the population and is most prevalent in women, with the highest incidence in women more than 65 years of age.[17] The risk of developing RA is about 3 to 5 times higher in individuals with a positive family history, which implies genetic predisposition.[19]

Inflammatory Bowel Disease

IBD is an idiopathic autoimmune disorder that occurs in individuals with a genetic predisposition who are exposed to environmental factors that trigger an immune response.[20,21] Dysregulation in the immune response changes the composition of host intestinal microbiota, creating an imbalance that destroys the mucosa and allows microbiota to invade the intestinal epithelium.[20–22] It is characterized by chronic, intermittent inflammation of the intestinal tract and involves 2 major disorders: Crohn disease and ulcerative colitis.[20,22–25] Many of the clinical and pathologic features of Crohn disease and ulcerative colitis overlap, but there are also come unique distinctions between them (**Table 1**).[21,24] A small percentage (10%–15%) of patients lack the distinct pathologic characteristics for either disease, and in such cases the disease is labeled indeterminate colitis.[21]

With either form of IBD, patients experience periods of relapse and remission, with varying levels of intensity and severity.[21,24] The clinical presentation, disease severity, location, degree of colon involvement, and phenotype determine the subclass of Crohn disease and ulcerative colitis.[24] Individuals with IBD are at an increased risk for the development of malignancy.[21]

Table 1 Inflammatory bowel disease symptoms	
Symptoms Suggestive of Inflammatory Damage	**General/Systemic Symptoms of UC and CD**

• Diarrhea:
  ○ May contain mucus and/or blood
  ○ Nocturnal diarrhea
  ○ Incontinence
• Constipation:
  ○ May be the chief complaint in ulcerative proctitis
  ○ Obstipation with absence of flatus in cases of bowel obstruction
• Rectal pain, bleeding, and urgency
• Tenesmus
• Abdominal cramps and pain:
  ○ CD: right lower quadrant of the abdomen
  ○ UC: periumbilical or left lower quadrant if moderate to severe
• Nausea and vomiting may be present with either, but more common in CD than UC
	• Fever
	  ○ Low-grade fever often initial warning sign of a flare
	• Anorexia
	• Weight loss, especially with CD
	• Fatigue; related
	• Night sweats
	• Growth retardation (children)
	• Primary amenorrhea
	• Malaise
	• Arthralgias

Abbreviations: CD, Crohn disease; UC, ulcerative colitis.
Data from Rowe WA, Lichenstein GR. Medscape Web site. Inflammatory bowel disease. 2017. Available at: https://emedicine.medscape.com/article/179037-overview. Accessed March 15, 2017 and World Gastroenterology Organisation Global Guidelines. Inflammatory bowel disease. World Health Organization Web site. 2015. Available at: http://www.worldgastroenterology.org/guidelines/global-guidelines/inflammatory-bowel-disease-ibd/inflammatory-bowel-disease-ibd-english. Accessed March 18, 2018.

The genetic risk for IBD varies among populations, and it is most prevalent among individuals of European descent.[23,25] The familial risk among individuals of African American, Asian, and Middle Eastern descent is lower; however, in newly industrialized and high-income countries, including areas in Asia, Africa, Canada, Australia, and New Zealand, there has been a steady increase in the incidence of IBD.[23–25] The incidence of Crohn disease in North America ranges from 3.1 to 20.2 cases per 100,000, and for ulcerative colitis the incidence ranges from 2.2 to 19.2 cases per 100,000.[24]

The hallmark of Crohn disease is transmural granulomatous inflammation and patches of skip lesions in different areas of the GI tract.[21,24] Inflammation may involve any segment of the GI tract from the mouth to the anus, but the most commonly affected areas are the ileum and proximal colon.[21,24] The transmural nature of Crohn disease means that it may involve several complications, including colon microperforations, strictures, fistulae, and obstructions, which usually do not occur with ulcerative colitis.[24]

Ulcerative colitis is characterized by inflammation that is limited to the intestinal mucosa, most often involves the rectum, and typically progresses proximally and in a continuous manner to other parts of the colon.[21,24] The location and degree of inflammation are used to characterize ulcerative colitis (**Box 1**).[21,24]

Systemic Lupus Erythematosus

SLE is a chronic multisystem autoimmune disease that involves inflammation of the skin, joints, kidneys, brain, and other organs.[26–28] Disease activity varies and is classified according to 1 of 3 patterns:

Box 1
Classification of ulcerative colitis

Type and definition

- Ulcerative proctitis
  - Inflammation that is located only in the rectum

- Ulcerative proctosigmoiditis
  - Inflammation involving the rectum and sigmoid colon, but not the sigmoid colon

- Left-sided distal ulcerative colitis
  - Inflammation that extends proximally from the rectum to the splenic flexure

- Extensive colitis
  - Inflammation that extends proximal to the splenic flexure, but that does not involve the cecum

- Pancolitis
  - Inflammation that spreads throughout the colon to the cecum

Data from Peppercorn MA, Cheifetz AS. Definition, epidemiology, and risk factors in inflammatory bowel disease. 2018. Available at: https://www.uptodate.com/contents/definition-epidemiology-and-risk-factors-in-inflammatory-bowel-disease/print?csi=7a136a39-10fd-439f-86ee-e7fbd61b81 27&source=contentShare. Accessed March 18, 2018; and Rowe WA, Lichenstein GR. Medscape Web site. 2017. Available at: https://emedicine.medscape.com/article/179037-overview. Accessed March 18, 2018.

- Intermittent: characterized by flares and remission of disease, including periods of quiescence between relapses[28]
- Chronically active: characterized by patterns of organ involvement[28]
- Quiescent: disease is present but inactive[28]

The cause of SLE is not fully known, but a genetic component has been clearly identified.[26,27] The risk ratio is 8 to 29 times higher in siblings than in the general population, and there is a 10-times risk increase in disease concordance in identical twins.[26]

SLE is more common in women than in men, at a ratio of 7:1 to 15:1, and it may occur at any age, but it most often occurs in individuals between the ages of 15 and 44 years.[26–29] It is most often diagnosed in individuals of African American and Asian descent.[29] Prevalence of SLE is estimated to range from about 5.8 to 130 per 100,000 population or about 1.5 million cases.[28]

Multiple Sclerosis

MS is an idiopathic, chronic inflammatory disease of the central nervous system.[30–32] In MS, the myelin sheath is damaged, thus affecting communication between the brain and the body and causing physical disabilities, visual disturbances, cognitive dysfunction, fatigue, and pain.[30–32] During the initial phase of the disease, inflammation is fleeting and temporary remyelination occurs, leading to episodes of recovery from neurologic dysfunction.[30,31] The physical, mental, and sociologic limitations caused by MS adversely affect quality of life.[31] MS occurs in individuals with a genetic predisposition who are exposed to environmental triggers.[30]

It is the second most common debilitating disease in young adults, and it is also one of the costliest chronic diseases in the Unites States.[31] MS can occur at any age, but it is usually diagnosed in individuals between the ages of 15 and 45 years.[31,32] It is more common in women than in men.[31] The average age at diagnosis of MS in women is 29 years, and 31 years of age in men.[31,32] In the United States, estimates of prevalence range from 58 to 95 per 100,000 population; this represents about 400,000 diagnosed individuals.[32] However, because misdiagnosis is common, these estimates may not accurately affect the true prevalence of MS.[32]

DIAGNOSIS

Clinical presentation and diagnosis of autoimmune disorders is disease specific and often corresponds with the degree of inflammation, as well as the systems involved.[1,6] A comprehensive history is essential in diagnosing all autoimmune disorders. In general, diagnosis of immune disorders is made based on a combination of clinical features, laboratory findings, and imaging results.[33]

Autoimmune Thyroid Disorders

HT is diagnosed based on clinical presentation of hypothyroidism, serum thyroid laboratory results demonstrating an increased TSH level, and thyroid ultrasonography results.[13,15,32] The onset of hypothyroidism is typically insidious, and the presentation may be subclinical, often detected after routine thyroid screening.[13,15,32]

Symptoms are usually nonspecific, except in the case of long-term and severe hypothyroidism presenting as myxedema coma, which is caused by an infectious state or major stressor.[32] Presenting symptoms are nonspecific and may include the following common complaints: fatigue, constipation, dry skin, and weight gain.[13,32] Other clinical features associated with HT include anemia, cold intolerance, bradycardia, bradypnea, hypoxia, sleep apnea, and menstrual irregularities.[13,32]

Physical examination findings depend on many factors, including the extent of hypothyroidism.[32] Patients with HT often present with an enlarged, firm, and rubbery thyroid gland. However, a normal or nonpalpable thyroid may also be present.[32] Other findings may include dry, brittle nails; paresthesias; and diminished deep tendon reflexes.[32] Laboratory and other diagnostic tests are also critical in the diagnosis of HT (**Table 2**). The approach to diagnosis of HT must include consideration that a small percentage (up to 15%) of elderly patients may present with increased TSH and normal free T4 levels, indicating subclinical hypothyroidism.[32] Patients who present with normal TSH levels and positive thyroid autoantibodies should have follow-up at least every 6 to 12 months to monitor symptoms and reevaluate serum thyroid and cholesterol levels for initiation of treatment.[32]

Although GD is classified as an organ-specific autoimmune disease, it can affect other organs, such as the eyes, skin, and joints.[12,34] Symptoms of thyrotoxicosis are the most common clinical presentation. In general, symptom onset is gradual, and patients seek a provider with complaints of fatigue, nervousness, insomnia, tachycardia, palpitations, and weight loss (despite polyphagia).[12,34] In addition, women may report metrorrhagia, and men often report decreased libido, erectile dysfunction, and gynecomastia.[12] Elderly patients may present with less severe symptoms.[12] The most common symptoms in the elderly population are apathy and lethargy, referred to as pathetic thyrotoxicosis.[12]

Specific clinical features of GD may include 1 or more of the following:

- Ophthalmopathy: inflammation and enlargement of the orbital tissues, resulting in exophthalmos[12]
- Goiter: abnormal enlargement of the thyroid gland[12]
- Onycholysis: painless separation of the nail from the nailbed[34]

Physical examination findings with GD vary and depend on many factors, including gender, the extent of hyperthyroidism, and age.[12,34] As with HT, in addition to clinical presentation, laboratory and other diagnostic tests are also critical in the diagnosis of

Table 2
Autoimmune disease diagnostic work-up

Disease Type	Diagnostic Work-up
Autoimmune thyroid disorders • HT • GD	• HT: thyroid panel (TSH, free T4, T3), thyroid autoantibodies (anti-TPO, anti-Tg), thyroid ultrasonography[13,32] • HT complication evaluation: CBC, CMP, total and fractionated lipid panel, CK, prolactin, CXR, ECG, echocardiogram[32] • GD: ultrasensitive thyrotropin assays, free T4 or T4 index, T3, LFTs, CBC, fasting lipid panel, HgA1c[34]
RA	• Laboratory tests: ESR, CRP, CBC, RF, ANA, anti-CCP, anti-MCV[33] • Imaging: radiographs, MRI, US[33]

IBD
• CD
• UC
	• CD:
	  ○ Laboratory tests: CBC, CMP, CRP, ESR, ASCA, p-ANCA, stool samples (WBCs, occult blood, ova and parasites, c-diff)[33]
	  ○ Imaging: CT, MRI, upper GI, colonoscopy, CT enterography, MR enterography[35]
	• UC:
	  ○ Labs: CBC, CMP, ESR, CRP, p-ANCA, stool samples (WBCs, occult blood, ova & parasites, c-diff)[36]
	  ○ Imaging: US, colonoscopy, CT, MRI[36]

SLE	• Laboratory tests: CBC, serum creatinine, ESR or CRP, LFTs, CK, complement levels, autoantibodies (multiple tests), UA with microscopy[26] • Complication evaluation: echocardiogram, MRI of the brain, joint effusion studies, CSF studies[26]
MS	• MRI of the brain and spinal cord, CSF studies[32] • Bloodwork: usually normal; used for exclusion of other conditions; ie, rheumatologic conditions, Lyme disease, syphilis, endocrine conditions, vitamin B_{12} deficiency, sarcoidosis, vasculitis[37]

This is a snapshot of the most commonly ordered tests. It is not an exhaustive list and should not be used as a guideline or screening tool for diagnosis of any of the listed autoimmune diseases.

Abbreviations: ANA, antinuclear antibody; ASCA, anti-*Saccharomyces cerevisiae* antibodies; CBC, complete blood count; CCP; citrullinated protein; c-diff, *Clostridium difficile*; CK, creatine kinase; CMP, complete metabolic profile; CRP, C-reactive protein; CSF, cerebrospinal fluid; CT, computed tomography; CXR, chest radiograph; ECG, electrocardiogram; ESR, erythrocyte sedimentation rate; HgA1c, hemoglobin A1c; LFT, liver function test; MCV, mean corpuscular volume; MR, magnetic resonance; p-ANCA, perinuclear antineutrophil cytoplasmic antibodies; RF, rheumatoid factor; Tg, thyroglobulin; TPO, thyroid peroxidase; UA, urinalysis; US, ultrasonography; WBCs, white blood cells.

Data from Refs.[21,26,32–34,37,45–47]

GD (see **Table 1**). The gold standard for diagnosis of thyrotoxicosis is measurement of free T3 and free T4 levels.[12] Increased total serum T3 and T4 levels with undetectable TSH levels is the hallmark of GD laboratory findings.[12]

Rheumatoid arthritis
Patients with RA typically present with hallmark clinical features of persistent, symmetric polyarthritis of the hands and feet. However, inflammation may affect any joint with a synovial membrane.[19,33] Because of its insidious onset, patients may initially report systemic and/or constitutional symptoms, such as low-grade fever, malaise, arthralgia, morning stiffness, fatigue, and weight loss, which usually occur before inflammation manifests.[33] Severity varies but, in patients with chronic RA, the disease progresses and causes joint destruction and deformity, leading to substantial

deterioration in physical functioning.[33] As a result, patients often complain of difficulty performing activities that require use of the hands and feet, such as personal hygiene, getting dressed, walking, standing, and other activities of daily living.[19,33]

Physical examination of patients with RA should include assessment of extra-articular manifestations (ie, vasculitis and interstitial lung disease), along with a thorough musculoskeletal assessment for the following[19,33]:

- Range of motion (ROM): limitations, stiffness, pain
- Tenderness
- Swelling
- Deformities
- Rheumatoid nodules

The expected findings in the joints are inflammation and swelling, warmth, tenderness, and decreased ROM.[33] Interosseous muscle atrophy of the hands, tenosynovitis, periarticular and generalized osteoporosis, and carpal tunnel syndrome are other common assessment findings.[33]

There are 3 categories of laboratory tests (see **Table 1**) with potential usefulness in diagnosing RA: (1) inflammatory makers, (2) hematologic parameters, and (3) immunologic parameters.[33] Increased erythrocyte sedimentation rate (ESR) and C-reactive protein (CRP) levels are inflammatory markers that indicate active disease.[19,34] A complete blood count (CBC) may reveal the presence of anemia of chronic disease and thrombocytosis.[33] Autoantibodies such as rheumatoid factor (RF), anti–citrullinated protein, and antinuclear antibody are the immunologic parameters used in the diagnosis of RA.[33]

Inflammatory Bowel Disease

The diagnosis of IBD is often delayed for months to years because patients present vague symptoms such as abdominal cramping, irregular bowel patterns, and mucus in stools.[21] The signs and symptoms of IBD correspond with the affected area of the intestinal tract and include manifestations directly related to inflammation and general/systemic symptoms (see **Table 2**).[21,35] When evaluating patients with signs and symptoms of IBD, the following must also be considered:

- Family history of IBD, colorectal cancer, and celiac disease
- Medication use: antibiotics and nonsteroidal antiinflammatory drugs (NSAIDs)
- Mood disorders
- Tobacco use
- Recent travel

At present, there are no laboratory tests available to provide a definitive diagnosis of IBD, although some tests provide supporting data useful for the management of IBD through the evaluation of nutritional status and vitamin and mineral deficiencies (see **Table 1**).[21] A CBC provides valuable data related to the following[21]:

- Anemia: acute or chronic blood loss, malabsorption, or chronic disease state
  - Mean corpuscular volume
    - Normal = anemia of chronic disease
    - Low = iron deficiency anemia (confirm with a serum total iron-binding capacity)
- Vitamin deficiency
  - B_{12} in patients with Crohn disease
- Leukocytosis (active inflammation)

ESR and CRP are not specific inflammatory markers for IBD, but they are useful in monitoring disease activity and evaluating response to treatment.[21] However, some patients with IBD have normal ESR and CRP levels, even in the presence of active inflammation.[21]

Systemic Lupus Erythematosus

In women of childbearing age, the hallmark presentation of SLE is a triad of fever, joint pain, and rash.[26,29] When patients present with these symptoms, prompt evaluation should be initiated.[26,29] Patients may also exhibit symptoms that manifest in any the following systems[26]:

- Constitutional: fatigue (most common constitutional symptom), fever, arthralgia, and changes in weight
- Cardiac: pericarditis
- Pulmonary: pleuritic pain possibly leading to chest pain and pleural effusion
- Renal: chronic and end-stage renal disease
- GI: nausea, dyspepsia, occasional abdominal pain
- Dermatologic: includes 3 American College of Rheumatology (ACR) diagnostic criteria for lupus[36]:
  - Malar rash: erythematous over the cheeks and nasal bridge (not the nasolabial folds); may be painful or pruritic, lasts days to weeks.
  - Photosensitivity: may be acute or chronic; usually lasts about 2 days.
  - Discoid lupus: characterized by a plaquelike appearance with follicular scarring that often appears after exposure to the sun.
- Musculoskeletal: symmetric, polyarticular joint pain, myalgia; symmetric or asymmetrical arthralgia and arthritis; swan neck deformities.
- Hematologic: history of leukopenia, lymphopenia, anemia, or thrombocytopenia.
- Neuropsychiatric: list of 19 symptoms, including seizure, psychosis, anxiety disorder, and acute confusional state.[26,36] A family history of autoimmune disease further increases the need to pursue a diagnosis of SLE.[26] Because patients with SLE are considered immunocompromised and have a greater risk of developing infection and complications, infection should always be ruled out.[26]

Changes in laboratory test results aid in diagnosis of acute or active SLE[26]:

- CBC: screening for cytopenia
- Creatinine and urinalysis: evaluating renal function
- ESR: may be increased with a normal CRP
- CRP: when increased with ESR, suspect infection

In general, CRP levels fluctuate during acute illness, whereas ESR lags.[26] In active SLE, complement levels (C3 and C4) may be decreased, and liver function tests (LFTs) may be mildly increased.[26] LFTs may also be increased as a result of medication response (ie, NSAIDs or azathioprine).[26] Several autoantibodies are measured for diagnosis of SLE but are not discussed in detail here (see **Table 1**). In certain circumstances, as indicated by clinical findings and laboratory studies, radiologic studies such as radiographs, echocardiography, and brain MRI, are used to evaluate and/or monitor disease progression and assess for complications, such as periarticular osteopenia, interstitial lung disease, pneumonitis, pulmonary emboli, pericardial effusion, pulmonary hypertension, lupus-related changes in white matter, vasculitis, and stroke.[26]

Multiple Sclerosis

Early diagnosis and treatment of MS are important to decrease disability and prevent relapses.[37] Use of the 2010 McDonald Criteria for diagnosis has resulted in earlier diagnosis of MS, with a high degree of specificity and sensitivity, enhancing opportunities for counseling patients and initiating treatment sooner.[37,38]

MS is diagnosed based on clinical features in combination with diagnostic testing.[37,38] Clinical presentation of MS may vary, but exacerbations usually manifest as central nervous system (CNS) symptoms that occur at different times and affect different parts of the body.[37,38] Patients may initially present with symptoms that manifest in the upper extremities, and, months later, return with complaints of symptoms affecting another part of the body.[37] When considering a diagnosis of MS, note that the symptoms must last longer than 24 hours.[37]

The classic presentation for patients with MS includes an extensive list of symptoms, ranging from early/initial onset to those that occur later in the disease process (**Box 2**).[37]

Of note, the progression of physical and cognitive decline may occur without the presence of clinical symptoms.[37] MRI of the CNS and cerebrospinal fluid analysis are the diagnostic tests used to support the diagnosis of MS.[37,38] Cerebrospinal fluid evaluation is typically negative except in cases of aseptic meningitis, vasculitis, and transverse myelitis.[39] Laboratory blood tests are used to exclude other conditions (see **Table 1**).[37,38]

TREATMENT AND CLINICAL MANAGEMENT

Treatment of autoimmune diseases is varied and is guided by the specific disease, its stage of presentation, and the symptoms experienced by the patient.[1,6] The primary goal of treatment, however, is always to decrease inflammation, minimize symptoms, and lessen the potential for relapse.[6] These comprehensive goals of treatment are focused on:

- Reduction or alleviation of symptoms[1]
- Controlling the autoimmune process[1]
- Remission induction
- Preventing or limiting disability

Hashimoto Thyroiditis

The primary treatment of a chronic autoimmune thyroiditis, such as Hashimoto thyroiditis, is focused on thyroid replacement.[40] This treatment is routinely performed through the prescription of thyroid prohormone (T4), which the body then converts to T3 to be used by the body. Monitoring of hormone levels should initially occur every 3 to 6 weeks, and medication titration should be performed based on TSH levels and symptom presentation.[40]

Rheumatoid Arthritis

When determining treatment options for RA, the following should be considered[41]:

- Extent of disease activity
- Comorbid conditions
- Stage of therapy

The 2 predominate pharmacologic classes used for treatment of RA are[41]:

- Rapid-acting antiinflammatories: NSAIDs or systemic versus intraarticular steroids
- Disease-modifying anti-rheumatic drugs (DMARDs): biologic or nonbiologic

---

Box 2
Classic multiple sclerosis symptoms

CNS-related symptoms

- Sensory loss: commonly paresthesias, which are usually an early complaint
- Symptoms associated with partial acute transverse myelitis
- Spinal cord motor symptoms: muscle cramping as a result of spasticity
- Spinal cord autonomic symptoms: bladder, bowel, and sexual dysfunction
- Cerebellar symptoms:
  - Charcot triad: dysarthria (scanning speech), nystagmus, and intention tremor
- Optic neuritis
- Trigeminal neuralgia: may occur as bilateral facial weakness or as trigeminal neuralgia
- Facial myokymia: irregular facial muscle twitching, which may occur as an initial symptom
- Eye symptoms: occur in 33% of patients, and may include diplopia on lateral gaze
- Heat intolerance
- Constitutional symptoms:
  - Fatigue: occurs in 70% of cases; although fatigue and depression may coexist, the two must be differentiated
  - Dizziness
  - Insomnia
  - Exertional exhaustion secondary to disability
- Pain: occurs in 30% to 50% of patients at some point

Neuropsychological

- Subjective cognitive difficulties:
  - Decreased attention span
  - Impaired concentration
  - Difficulty with memory
  - Impaired judgment
- Depression
- Euphoria (not as common as depression)
- Bipolar disorder or frank dementia: may appear late in the disease process but can occur at the time of initial diagnosis

Data from Luzzio C, Dagond F. Multiple sclerosis. Medscape Web site. 2017. Available at: https://emedicine.medscape.com/article/1146199-overview. Accessed March 18, 2018.

Before the initiation of DMARD therapy, a complete screening for hepatitis B and C should be completed. In addition, laboratory screenings should be performed of ESR, CRP, CBC, creatinine, LFTs, and tuberculosis. Screening for antimalarial toxicity should also be performed to aid in dosage guidelines for nonbiologic DMARDs.[41]

Inflammatory Bowel Disease

The goal for treatment of IBD is to control inflammation, which can be approached through the use of antiinflammatory agents (NSAIDs or steroids), monoclonal antibodies, or immunosuppressive agents. Antidiarrheal agents may also be used to help control symptoms. Which course of treatment is chosen is highly dependent on whether the patient is experiencing ulcerative colitis or Crohn disease. In addition, the stage of disease is a significant contributor in the decision-making process.[22,42]

Systemic Lupus Erythematosus

Numerous nonpharmacologic measures have been found to have an impact on the frequency and severity of SLE flares. These include sun exposure, diet and nutrition, exercise, and smoking. When deciding to initiate pharmacologic management, the choice of therapy is highly individualized and depends on the predominant symptoms, organ involvement, response to previous therapy, and disease activity and severity. Similar to the treatment of RA, the use of antimalarial agents is highly recommended. Additional therapies, such as NSAIDs, prednisone, or immunosuppressive agents, depends on the severity of the disease and the combination of manifestations.[43]

Multiple Sclerosis

Progressive MS is more difficult to manage than patients who present with an MS relapse. The treatment options for progressive MS are focused on the use of immunosuppressive therapies, such as interferon, biologic agents, and monoclonal antibodies. The use of nonspecific immunosuppressants has shown good short-term control of progressive MS. However, poor long-term results have been seen. Pulse doses of intravenous glucocorticoids are recommended for primary progressive MS as well as relapsing-remitting MS.[44]

PROGNOSIS

Prognosis is unique to the disease and systems involved.[1] As with all chronic diseases, positive health outcomes are based on a multitude of variables. In general, early and accurate diagnosis, timely initiation of treatment, patient compliance with the management plan, and appropriate follow-up directly affect health outcomes.

Patients with Hashimoto thyroiditis have an excellent prognosis with early diagnosis and treatment and meticulous follow-up.[32] However, a poor prognosis and high mortality is associated with patients with untreated myxedema coma.[32] After surgical induction of hypothyroidism, most patients do well with replacement therapy.[34] The ophthalmopathy also becomes inactive.[34] Occasionally, even after a thyroidectomy, some thyroid tissue may remain and require further surgery or ablation with radioactive iodine.[34]

RA is characterized by periods of exacerbation and remission, and the prognosis depends on several factors, including timing of diagnosis, initiation of and response to treatments, and disease complications.[33] In some patients, RA is self-limited and in others it is chronic and progressive, making the prognosis individualized.[33] In general, patients with positive RF results have a much worse prognosis than those with negative RF results.[33] Individuals with short-term exacerbations and spontaneous remission have a better prognosis.[33]

The prognosis for individuals with IBD is largely based on the form of IBD: Crohn versus ulcerative colitis.[21] The mortality is higher in patients with Crohn disease than in those with ulcerative colitis, because individuals with ulcerative colitis have the same mortality as the general population.[21] IBD increases the risk of small bowel malignancy in patients with Crohn disease, and patients with pancolitis (a form of ulcerative colitis) have a risk of colon cancer after 8 to 10 years of having the disease.[21]

Based on disease severity and systems affected, the prognosis for SLE is unique to individual patients.[26] SLE varies from benign to fatal, and the survival rate is higher when the disease is limited to the integumentary and musculoskeletal systems.[26] In individuals with renal and CNS involvement, the prognosis is worse.[26] Because of earlier diagnosis, advances in treatment options, and improvements in medical care, mortality associated with SLE has decreased.[26] Despite these improvements, most (35%) SLE-related deaths occur among the young to middle-aged adult population, specifically in patients younger than 45 years of age.[26]

The prognosis for individuals with MS is largely based on treatment. Significant disability occurs within 20 to 25 years after disease onset in more than 30% of those who do not receive treatment.[37] Although several disease-modifying agents have slowed the progression of MS in research trials, long-term prevention of disability is unknown.[37] Men with primary progressive MS rapidly develop disability because of limited response to treatment, and this ultimately contributes to these patients having the worst prognosis.[37] There is only a slight decrease in the life expectancy of patients with MS, with death most often associated with secondary complications from renal or pulmonary causes.[37]

SUMMARY

Identification and management of immunosuppressive/immunocompromised syndromes continues to be an area of difficulty, from diagnosis to management and treatment. Active research continues to better delineate pharmacologic agents that specifically target the disease pathways of many of these syndromes, numbering greater than 100. Knowledge deficit continues to create an additive complexity to the medical community's ability to effectively manage autoimmune syndromes. It is because of this lack of awareness of both the American public and the medical community that providers do not think to ask, and patients do not think to share, the presence of a family history of autoimmune disorders.[3]

The use of biologic agents that modify specific inflammatory effector pathways continues to be a growing and efficient pharmacologic approach.[5] Research to further develop medications that will completely reverse, if not cure, these diseases provides hope for possible modification of the host immune system to restore balance and immune tolerance to the human body.

REFERENCES

1. NIH/US National Library of Medicine. Medline Plus Medical Encyclopedia Web site. Autoimmune disorders. Available at: https://medlineplus.gov/ency/article/000816.htm. Accessed March 2, 2018.

2. Fairweather D, Rose NR. Women and autoimmune diseases. Emerg Infect Dis 2004;10(11):2005–11.

3. American Autoimmune Related Diseases Association. The cost burden of autoimmune disease: the latest front in the war on healthcare spending. Eastpointe (MI): American Autoimmune Related Diseases Association; 2011. Available at: http://www.diabetesed.net/page/_files/autoimmune-diseases.pdf.

4. Hayter SM, Cook MC. Updated assessment of the prevalence, spectrum, and case definition of autoimmune disease. Autoimmun Rev 2012;11(10):754–65.

5. Wang L, Wang F, Gershwin ME. Human autoimmune diseases: a comprehensive update. J Intern Med 2015;278:369–95.

6. National Institute of Arthritis and Musculoskeletal and Skin Disease. Understanding autoimmune diseases. 2016. Available at: https://www.niams.nih.gov/sites/default/files/catalog/files/understanding_autoimmune.pdf. Accessed March 1, 2018.

7. Autoimmune Disease. National Institutes of Health Web site. Available at: https://www.niams.nih.gov/health-topics/autoimmune-diseases/advanced. Accessed March 1, 2018.

8. Lu M, Taylor BV, Körner H. Genomic effects of the vitamin D receptor: potentially the link between vitamin D, immune cells, and multiple sclerosis. Front Immunol 2018;9:477.

9. Vojdani A, Pollard KM, Campbell AW. Environmental triggers and autoimmunity. Autoimmune Dis 2014;798029:1–2.

10. Takaba H, Hiroshi T. The mechanisms of T cell selection in the thymus. Trends Immunol 2017;805–16. https://doi.org/10.1016/j.it.2017.07.010.

11. Antonelli A, Ferrari SM, Corrado AD, et al. Autoimmune thyroid disorders. Autoimmun Rev 2015;14:174–80.

12. Menconi F, Marocci C, Marino M. Diagnosis and classification of Graves' disease. Autoimmun Rev 2014;13:398–402.

13. Caturegli P, Remigis AD, Rose NR. Hashimoto thyroiditis: clinical and diagnostic criteria. Autoimmun Rev 2014;13:391–7.

14. Hashimoto's disease. Mayo clinic Web site. Available at: https://www.mayoclinic.org/diseases-conditions/hashimotos-disease/symptoms-causes/syc-20351855. Accessed March 1, 2018.

15. Davies TF. Pathogenesis of Hashimoto's thyroiditis (chronic autoimmune thyroiditis). UpToDate Web site. 2018. Available at: https://www.uptodate.com/contents/pathogenesis-of-hashimotos-thyroiditis-chronic-autoimmune-thyroiditis?csi=8cc8c97b-e5ba-489f-ac93-1c9070caab2a&source=contentShare. Accessed March 1, 2018.

16. Davies TF. Pathogenesis of Graves' disease. UpToDate Web site. 2018. Available at: https://www.uptodate.com/contents/pathogenesis-of-graves-disease?csi=5288a9d0-0fd1-409b-8e85-170f57f63c93&source=contentShare. Accessed March 1, 2018.

17. Scott DL, Wolfe F, Huizinga TW. Rheumatoid arthritis. Lancet 2010;376:1094–108.

18. Moreland LW, Cannella A. General principles of management of rheumatoid arthritis in adults. UpToDate Web site. 2018. Available at: https://www.uptodate.com/contents/general-principles-of-management-of-rheumatoid-arthritis-in-adults?csi=1c14350a-55a4-4b68-a25b-46aa5ed073af&source=contentShare. Accessed March 1, 2018.

19. Smolen JS, Aletaha D, McInnes IB. Rheumatoid arthritis. Lancet 2016;388(10055):2023–38.

20. Molodecky NA, Soon IS, Rabi DM, et al. Increasing incidence and prevalence of the inflammatory bowel diseases with time, based on systematic review. Gastroenterology 2012;142(1):46.

21. Rowe WA, Lichenstein GR. Medscape Web site. Inflammatory bowel disease. 2017. Available at: https://emedicine.medscape.com/article/179037-overview. Accessed March 15, 2017.

22. Ramos de Mattos BR, Garcia MPG, Nogueira JB, et al. Inflammatory bowel disease: an overview of immune mechanisms and biological treatments. Mediators Inflamm 2015;493012:1–11.

23. Kaplan GG, Ng SC. Understanding and preventing the global increase of inflammatory bowel disease. Gastroenterology 2017;125:313321.

24. Peppercorn MA, Cheifetz AS. Definition, epidemiology, and risk factors in inflammatory bowel disease. 2018. Available at: https://www.uptodate.com/contents/definition-epidemiology-and-risk-factors-in-inflammatory-bowel-disease/print?csi=7a136a39-10fd-439f-86ee-e7fbd61b8127&source=contentShare. Accessed March 1, 2018.

25. Ng SC, Shi HY, Hamidi N, et al. Worldwide incidence and prevalence of inflammatory bowel disease in the 21st century: a systematic review of population-based studies. Lancet 2017;390:2769–78.

26. Bartels CN, Muller D. Systemic lupus erythematosus. Medscape Web site. 2017. Available at: https://emedicine.medscape.com/article/332244-overview#a3. Accessed March 3, 2018.

27. Gordon C, Amissah-Arthur MB, Gayed M, et al. The British Society for Rheumatology guideline for the management of systemic lupus erythematosus in adults. Rheumatology (Oxford) 2018;57(1):e1.

28. Wallace DJ. Overview of the management and prognosis of systemic lupus erythematosus in adults. UpToDate Web site. 2018. Available at: https://www.uptodate.com/contents/overview-of-the-clinical-manifestations-of-systemic-lupus-erythematosus-in-adults?csi=d423d8fe-4d14-4827-b211-921416724a41&source=contentShare. Accessed March 5, 2018.

29. NIH/US National Library of Medicine. Medline Plus Medical Encyclopedia Web site. Systemic lupus erythematosus. 2018. Available at: https://medlineplus.gov/ency/article/000435.htm. Accessed March 17, 2018.

30. Compston A, Coles A. Multiple sclerosis. Lancet 2008;372(9648):1502–17.

31. Wingerchuk DM, Carter JL. Multiple sclerosis: current and emerging disease-modifying therapies and treatment strategies. Mayo Clin Proc 2014;89(2):225–40.

32. Lee SL, Nagelberg SB, Odeke S. Hashimoto thyroiditis. Medscape Web site. 2018. Available at: https://emedicine.medscape.com/article/120937-overview#a6. Accessed March 17, 2018.

33. Smith HR, Brown A. Rheumatoid arthritis. Medscape Web site. 2018. Available at: https://emedicine.medscape.com/article/331715-overview#a6. Accessed March 17, 2018.

34. Yeung SJ, Habra MA, Chiu AC. Graves disease. Medscape Web site. 2017. Available at: https://emedicine.medscape.com/article/120619-overview#a2. Accessed March 17, 2018.

35. World Gastroenterology Organisation Global Guidelines. Inflammatory bowel disease. World Health Organization Web site. Published 2015. Available at: http://www.worldgastroenterology.org/guidelines/global-guidelines/inflammatory-bowel-disease-ibd/inflammatory-bowel-disease-ibd-english. Accessed March 18, 2018.

36. Karlson M, Khoshbin S, Rogers M. The American College of Rheumatology nomenclature and case definitions for neuropsychiatric lupus syndromes. Arthritis Rheum 1999;42(4):599–608.

37. Luzzio C, Dagond F. Multiple sclerosis. Medscape Web site. 2017. Available at: https://emedicine.medscape.com/article/1146199-overview. Accessed March 17, 2018.

38. Polman CH, Reingold SC, Banwell B, et al. Diagnostic criteria for multiple sclerosis: 2010 revisions to the McDonald criteria. Ann Neurol 2011;69(2):292–302.

39. Schur PH. Diagnostic approach to the neuropsychiatric manifestations of systemic lupus erythematosus. In: Aminoff MJ, Silver JM, Wilterdink JL, et al, editors. UpToDate. Waltham (MA): UpToDate; 2018. Available at: https://www.uptodate.com/contents/diagnostic-approach-to-the-neuropsychiatric-manifestations-of-systemic-lupus-erythematosus. Accessed March 28, 2018.

40. Ross DS. Treatment of primary hypothyroidism in adults. In: Cooper DS, Mulder JE, editors. UpToDate. Waltham (MA): UpToDate; 2018. Available at: https://www.uptodate.com/contents/treatment-of-primary-hypothyroidism-in-adults. Accessed March 28, 2018.

41. Moreland LW, Cannella A. General principles of management of rheumatoid arthritis in adults. In: O'Dell JR, Romain PL, editors. UpToDate. Waltham (MA): UpToDate; 2018. Available at: https://www.uptodate.com/contents/general-principles-of-management-of-rheumatoid-arthritis-in-adults. Accessed March 28, 2018.

42. Fakhoury M, Negrulj R, Mooranian A, et al. Inflammatory bowel disease: clinical aspects and treatments. J Inflamm Res 2014;7:113–20.

43. Wallace DJ. Overview of the management and prognosis of systemic lupus erythematosus in adults. In: Pisetsky DS, Schur PH, Ramirez Curtis M, editors. UpToDate. Waltham (MA): UpToDate; 2018. Available at: https://www.uptodate.com/contents/overview-of-the-management-and-prognosis-of-systemic-lupus-erythematosus-in-adults. Accessed March 28, 2018.

44. Olek MJ. Treatment of progressive multiple sclerosis in adults. In: González-Scarano F, Dashe JF, editors. UpToDate. Waltham (MA): UpToDate; 2018. Available at: https://www.uptodate.com/contents/treatment-of-progressive-multiple-sclerosis-in-adults. Accessed March 28, 2018.

45. NIH/US National Library of Medicine. Multiple sclerosis. Medline Plus Medical Encyclopedia Web site. 2018. Available at: https://medlineplus.gov/multiplesclerosis.html. Accessed March 17, 2018.

46. Ghazi LJ. Crohn disease workup. Medscape Web site. 2017. Available at: https://emedicine.medscape.com/article/172940-workup#c9. Accessed March 18, 2018.

47. Basson MD. Ulcerative colitis workup. Medscape Web site. 2017. Available at: https://emedicine.medscape.com/article/183084-workup#c14. Accessed March 18, 2018.

Fat Embolism Syndrome

Lauren E. Fukumoto, MSN, AGACNP-BC, CNP, CCRN[a],*,
Kathryn D. Fukumoto, BSN, RN, CCRN[b]

KEYWORDS

- Fat embolism syndrome • Fat embolism • Long bone fractures • Trauma

KEY POINTS

- Fat embolism syndrome (FES) is most commonly associated with long bone fractures and orthopedic procedures involving the femur.
- The classic symptom triad includes respiratory insufficiency, neurologic dysfunction, and petechial rash.
- Currently there are no standardized diagnostic and clinical criteria for FES, and diagnosis is often based on exclusion because signs and symptoms are typically nonspecific.
- Management is primarily supportive. Respiratory and neurologic status should be monitored closely in patients who are at high risk, so therapeutic treatment may be initiated promptly.
- Appropriate patient resuscitation and early fracture fixation of long bones is an effective method to prevent or minimize the severity of FES.

INTRODUCTION
Definition

A fat embolism (FE) is defined as the presence of fat globules within the circulatory system, which may occur with or without clinical symptoms. These FEs most often collect in regions with abundant microvasculature, including the lungs (pulmonary FE) and brain (cerebral FE). FE syndrome (FES) is a defining set of clinical characteristics that result as a complication secondary to the presence of FE and are not always present in patients with FE.[1–3]

Incidence

The incidence of FE is much more frequent than the incidence of FES. FEs are present in almost all patients with fractures or traumatic injury, although few develop FES. The highest incidence of FES is in patients with traumatic injuries, in particular those with long bone fractures, at a rate of approximately 3% to 4%.[1,4] Surgical procedures

[a] Neurosurgery, Mount Carmel Health Systems, 6001 East Broad Street, Columbus, OH 43213, USA; [b] Neurosciences and Trauma Intensive Care Unit, John Muir Medical Center, 1601 Ygnacio Valley Road, Walnut Creek, CA 94598, USA
* Corresponding author.
E-mail address: laurenfukumoto@gmail.com

Nurs Clin N Am 53 (2018) 335–347
https://doi.org/10.1016/j.cnur.2018.04.003
0029-6465/18/© 2018 Elsevier Inc. All rights reserved.
nursing.theclinics.com

involving bones or disruption of fat, such as intramedullary nailing, arthroplasties, lipo-suction, and bone marrow harvesting,[4] are also highly associated with incidence of FES.

The incidence of FES varies widely depending on the type of study performed. Retrospective studies show the incidence of FES at less than 1%,[2,5,6] whereas pro-spective studies reflect a rate of 11% to 19%.[2] On autopsy of patients with fractures, 82% were found to have FEs, whereas only 33% of these patients with FE were found to have FES.[7] Criteria used to diagnose FES may also affect incidence. For example, hypoxemia may be a subclinical indicator for the development of FES and was found in 35% of patients with femur, tibia, or pelvis fractures.[7] Propofol and other lipid-based infusions are also associated with causing respiratory failure, which is a clinical feature of FES.[2]

Certain preexisting conditions may also contribute to the development of FES. Pa-tients with hereditary conditions, such as Duchenne muscular dystrophy,[8] were shown at higher risk for the development of FES on traumatic injury. Patients with sickle cell disease have a high incidence of nontraumatic FES due to bone marrow necrosis, 57% in 1 study done on autopsy.[9]

Overall, the incidence of FES is difficult to determine, because it is dependent on many variable factors. The criteria for diagnosis of FES is still poorly defined, subse-quently affecting the standardization of incidence.

PATHOPHYSIOLOGY

Although the exact mechanisms that result in FES are unknown, it is likely that both mechanical and biochemical components contribute to the pathologic and physical manifestations of FES (**Fig. 1**).

Mechanical Theory

The mechanical theory postulates that outside mechanical forces, such as traumatic injury or invasive surgery, cause FEs from bone marrow or adipose tissue to enter venous circulation. These emboli become lodged first in the pulmonary microvascula-ture,[11] leading to pulmonary dysfunction, but then can also occlude the microvascu-lature within other organ systems, causing multiorgan dysfunction.

It is unclear how FEs gain access to the arterial circulation. One theory suggests that increased pressure in the right heart physically forces fat globules through the capillary membranes and into arteries,[3] leading to systemic circulation and thus organ dysfunc-tion. The use of an echocardiogram supports this theory, allowing the visualization of embolic material passing into the left atrium.[12]

Some investigators theorize that a patent foramen ovale (PFO) may be an alternate mechanism through which FE are passed into arterial circulation.[1] Other studies, how-ever, suggest less of an emphasis on the role of a PFO and perhaps more focus on arteriovenous shunts and the role of systemic circulation of the lungs as a means of passing FEs into arterial circulation.[13]

Biochemical Theory

Although FES occurs most frequently in patients having sustained mechanical injury, cases of FES have been reported without mechanical forces at play, suggesting a biochemical component to the pathophysiology of this syndrome. Once FEs enter into venous circulation, they trigger a cascade of inflammatory and thrombotic events that lead to the rapid production of fibrin and aggregation of platelets.[3] Release of free fatty acids (FFAs) into circulation also stimulates the release of inflammatory

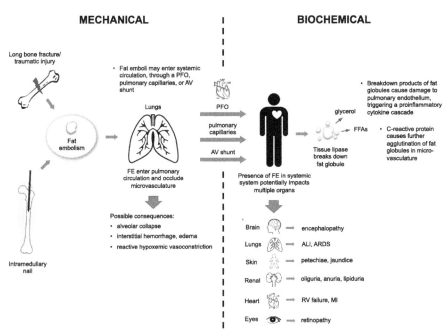

Fig. 1. Possible mechanisms that lead to FES. FEs enter venous circulation through traumatic injury or surgery and become lodged in the microvasculature of the lungs. FEs may then enter systemic circulation through a PFO, pulmonary capillaries, or an arteriovenous (AV) shunt and become lodged in the microvasculature of other organs, including the brain, kidneys, liver, and eyes, causing disruption of organ function and clinical manifestations of FES. Once in the bloodstream, it is theorized that tissue lipase breaks down the fat globules, and the breakdown products (FFAs and glycerol) trigger a proinflammatory cytokine cascade that causes further aggregation of fat globules throughout the vascular system as well as causing further damage to the lungs and other organs. MI, myocardial infarction; RV, right ventricle. (*Data from* Refs.[1–3,10])

mediators, such as C-reactive protein, which causes the aggregation of FFAs and resultant fat globules. This leads to symptoms of acute respiratory distress syndrome (ARDS), cardiac contractility dysfunction, and increase in plasma lipase concentration and can eventually lead to multiorgan dysfunction and failure.[10,11]

Specifically in the lungs, FFAs directly damage pulmonary endothelial cells, causing alveolar edema and possibly hemorrhage. Furthermore, this damage to lung tissue triggers activation of a proinflammatory cytokine cascade whose chemical mediators lead to vasculitis, pneumonitis, and hypoxia, which can progress to the development of acute lung injury (ALI), ARDS, and respiratory failure.[1–3,10]

CLINICAL PRESENTATION
Pulmonary

Respiratory abnormalities are the most common manifestation of FES and occur in up to 75% of patients.[10,14] Patients typically present with nonspecific respiratory derangements, such as hypoxemia, tachypnea, and dyspnea. These symptoms may manifest as early as 12 hours after initial insult.[1,3] Pulmonary symptoms can range from mild hypoxemia to respiratory failure requiring mechanical ventilation and typically peak after 48 hours to 72 hours. Respiratory failure can progress rapidly, and patients may develop ARDS.[3,14,15]

Neurologic

Central nervous system dysfunction is another common manifestation of FES, occurring in up to 86% of patients,[14] typically after the onset of respiratory symptoms. In the setting of FES, neurologic changes rarely occur in isolation. These symptoms are also nonspecific and may range from drowsiness, confusion, and restlessness to seizure and coma.[3] Focal deficits are less common but have been reported.[14] Fortunately, neurologic changes usually resolve.[2,3]

Petechial Rash

Petechial rash is the most characteristic symptom of FES,[2] although it occurs in only 20% to 60% of patients. The rash is most often located on nondependent areas of the body, such as the anterior chest, oral mucous membranes, conjunctiva, neck, and axillae.[3,14] Petechiae typically appear 24 hours to 48 hours after initial insult and usually resolve within 1 day to 7 days.[3,14]

Other Manifestations

Less common manifestations of FES include the following: fever, myocardial ischemia or infarction, cor pulmonale, hypotension, retinopathy, jaundice, oliguria or anuria, lipiduria, anemia, thrombocytopenia, coagulation abnormalities, and obstructive shock.[3,14] See **Table 1** for a summary of signs and symptoms.

DIAGNOSIS
Diagnostic Criteria

The diagnosis of FES is often one of exclusion, because clinical symptoms and laboratory and imaging findings associated with FES are typically nonspecific. At present, there are no standardized criteria that define FES. A combination of the Gurd and Wilson[16] and the Lindeque criteria,[17] however, is the most widely accepted diagnostic approach for FES.[3]

Gurd and Wilson[16] defined major features as respiratory insufficiency, cerebral involvement, and petechial rash. Minor features were defined as pyrexia, tachycardia, retinal changes, jaundice, and renal changes. Laboratory characteristics were defined as anemia, thrombocytopenia, elevated erythrocyte sedimentation rate, and fat macroglobulinemia. Patients with at least 1 major criteria, at least 4 minor criteria, and fat macroglobulinemia were defined as having FES.[16]

The Gurd and Wilson criteria, however, have been criticized for excluding arterial blood gas (ABG) results, because objective hypoxemia may be detected prior to the onset of any clinical symptoms. Lindeque and colleagues[17] suggested that, for patients with tibial and/or femur fractures, FES should be diagnosed if 1 or more of the following features were present: sustained Pao_2 less than 60 mm Hg, sustained $Paco_2$ greater than 55 mm Hg or pH less than 7.3, sustained respiratory rate greater than 35 breaths per minute after adequate sedation, and increased work of breathing (defined as dyspnea, accessory muscle use, and tachycardia) combined with anxiety. See **Table 2** for a summary of the diagnostic criteria.

Imaging

Chest radiograph
Chest radiograph (CXR) abnormalities are found in approximately 30% to 50% of patients with FES.[3,16] They are typically described as bilateral diffuse, patchy infiltrates.[14,16] In more severe cases, CXR may reveal airspace consolidations, which are associated with pulmonary edema and alveolar hemorrhage.[14] CXRs offer limited

Table 1
Fat embolism syndrome signs and symptoms

Body System	Signs and Symptoms
Pulmonary	Hypoxemia Tachypnea Dyspnea Rales Rhonchi Wheezing Pulmonary edema Respiratory failure ARDS
Neurologic	Drowsiness Confusion Disorientation Restlessness Seizure Stupor Coma Focal deficits
Dermatologic	Petechial rash
Cardiovascular	Increased pulmonary artery pressure Hypotension Decreased cardiac output Arrhythmias Right ventricular failure Cor pulmonale Obstructive shock Myocardial ischemia Myocardial infarction Cardiac arrest
Renal	Oliguria Anuria Lipiduria
Liver	Jaundice
Hematologic	Anemia Thrombocytopenia Coagulopathy Fat macroglobulinemia
Ophthalmologic	Retinopathy
Systemic	Fever

Data from Refs.[3,14,15]

diagnostic value because findings are nonspecific to FES and their appearance may lag behind clinical symptoms by 12 hours to 72 hours.[3,14] Serial CXRs, however, may be useful for monitoring disease progression[18] (**Fig. 2**).

Chest CT
Chest CT is considered the best imaging modality to evaluate for FES.[18] The most common chest CT abnormality found in patients with FES has been described as patchy, well-demarcated, ground-glass opacities. Small centrilobular nodules are a less common finding.[18] Airspace consolidations in more severe cases of FES and small bilateral pleural effusions have also been reported.[18] Several studies have

Table 2
Diagnostic criteria

Gurd and Wilson Criteria[16] Fat Embolism Syndrome if at Least 1 Major Criteria, at Least 4 Minor Criteria, and Fat Macroglobulinemia			Lindeque Criteria[17] Fat Embolism Syndrome if Tibia/Femur Fracture and 1 or More of the Following
Major Criteria	Minor Criteria	Laboratory Abnormalities	
Respiratory insufficiency	Pyrexia	Anemia	Pao_2 <60 mm Hg
Neurologic dysfunction	Tachycardia	Thrombocytopenia	$Paco_2$ >55
Petechial rash	Retinal changes	Elevated erythrocyte sedimentation rate	pH <7.3
	Jaundice	Fat macroglobulinemia	Respiratory rate >35 breaths per minute
	Renal changes		Increased work of breathing and anxiety

Data from Gurd AR, Wilson RI. The fat embolism syndrome. J Bone Joint Surg Br 1974;56(3):408–16; and Lindeque BG, Schoeman HS, Dommisee GF, et al. Fat embolism and the fat embolism syndrome. A double-blind therapeutic study. J Bone Joint Surg Br 1987;69(1):123–31.

suggested a direct correlation between the extent of lung involvement on chest CT imaging and severity of pulmonary symptoms (**Figs. 3** and **4**).

Brain MRI

Brain MRI is considered the most sensitive imaging modality to detect cerebral fat emboli.[18] Diffusion-weighted imaging may reveal a starfield appearance with multiple punctate, hyperintense foci that follow a watershed distribution.[18,19] These findings may be present as early as 1 hour after symptom onset. Other brain MRI abnormalities are more nonspecific and may include hypointense lesions on T1-weighted images and small, scattered hyperintense lesions involving both the gray matter and white matter on T2-weighted images.[18,19] Although the number and size of these lesions

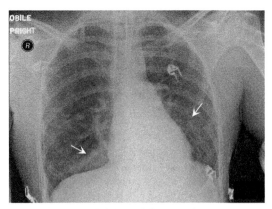

Fig. 2. FES in a 23-year-old-man with bilateral femoral fractures presenting with hypoxia and confusion. CXR demonstrates patchy, ill-defined opacities in the perihilar and lower lobe regions (*arrows*). These findings were monitored with plain radiographs and resolved completely in 1 week. (*From* Newbigin K, Souza CA, Torres C, et al. Fat embolism syndrome: state-of-the-art review focused on pulmonary imaging findings. Respir Med 2016;113:96; with permission.)

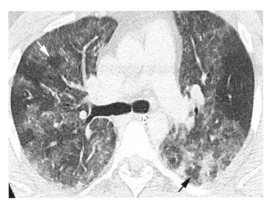

Fig. 3. A 19-year-old man presenting with pronounced hypoxia after femoral nail fixation 3 days after trauma, progressing to respiratory failure requiring respiratory and circulatory support. Axial HRCT image demonstrates diffuse ground-glass opacities with areas of lobular sparing (*arrow*). (*From* Newbigin K, Souza CA, Torres C, et al. Fat embolism syndrome: state-of-the-art review focused on pulmonary imaging findings. Respir Med 2016;113:97; with permission.)

are variable, they have been shown to correlate clinically with the extent of neurologic impairment (**Fig. 5**).

Ultrasound

Ultrasound can be used to detect emboli intraoperatively. Transesophageal echocardiogram (TEE) is used intraoperatively to identify and monitor embolic material in the right atrium in real time. TEE has 100% specificity and 80% sensitivity for emboli large enough to cause hemodynamic instability,[3] but embolic material often is only presumed to be fat. It is likely that these emboli are also made of bone and other marrow

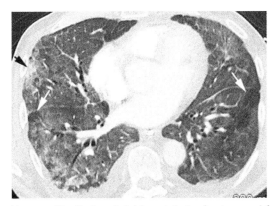

Fig. 4. A 67-year-old man with displaced right acetabular fracture and fracture-dislocation of the right hip secondary to a motor vehicle accident, presenting with acute respiratory failure 2 days after internal fixation of the fractures. Axial CT image demonstrates diffuse ground-glass opacities with areas of lobular sparing (*white arrows*) and small peripheral consolidation in the right middle lobe (*black arrow*). (*From* Newbigin K, Souza CA, Torres C, et al. Fat embolism syndrome: state-of-the-art review focused on pulmonary imaging findings. Respir Med 2016;113:97; with permission.)

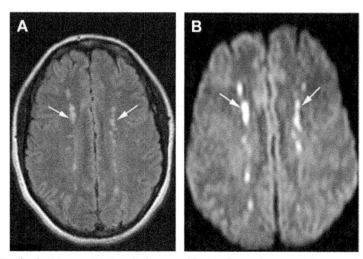

Fig. 5. Cerebral FE in a patient with decreased level of consciousness after a motor vehicle accident and femoral fracture. (*A*) Axial fluid-attenuated inversion recovery image of the brain demonstrates multiple tiny hyperintense foci distributed in a linear fashion along the centrum semiovale bilaterally (*arrows*). (*B*) Diffusion-weighted imaging, reveals multiple lesions of high signal intensity (*arrows*) in a watershed distribution, along the bilateral centrum semiovale, indicating restricted diffusion due to cytotoxic edema. (*From* Newbigin K, Souza CA, Torres C, et al. Fat embolism syndrome: state-of-the-art review focused on pulmonary imaging findings. Respir Med 2016;113:99; with permission.)

contents. Although FES cannot be definitively diagnosed by TEE, FES should be highly suspected in patients with echogenic evidence of right heart emboli and an associated decrease in Pao$_2$.[3] There have also been several studies that demonstrated the ability of transcranial Doppler to detect cerebral microemboli during orthopedic procedures.[12,20–22] These microemboli, however, were also not definitively determined to be fat.

Laboratory Tests

Although nonspecific, ABG analysis is the most useful laboratory test in the diagnosis of FES. Patients with FES often have a Pao$_2$ of less than 60 mm Hg, indicating hypoxemia. Bronchial alveolar lavage fluid containing more than 30% macrophages with lipid inclusions is highly suggestive of FES,[2,3] although it is still nonspecific, and collecting an adequate sample may not be possible or practical. Other laboratory tests are of limited diagnostic utility.

In the presences of FES, certain biochemical tests may reveal increased serum lipase and phospholipase A2. Cytologic examination of blood, urine, sputum, and cerebrospinal fluid may also show the presence of fat globules. These tests, however, are considered unreliable and nondiagnostic.[3] Hematologic studies may show anemia and thrombocytopenia. Other laboratory abnormalities associated with FES include elevated plasma FFA levels, hypocalcemia, and elevated levels of cortisol, glucagon, and catecholamines.[14]

MANAGEMENT

There are no definitive or specific treatments of FES; therefore, management is entirely supportive.

Pulmonary

Because FES may quickly progress to respiratory failure, early detection is important so that supportive treatment can be started promptly. In high-risk patients, respiratory status should be monitored closely via continuous pulse oximetry and ABG analysis, because these may detect oxygen desaturations prior to the onset of clinical symptoms.[23] Initial or mild FES is treated with supplemental oxygen, titrated to maintain normal Pao_2. FES that progresses to respiratory failure requires mechanical ventilation. Because respiratory failure due to FES is clinically indistinguishable from ALI and ARDS, ventilatory management is essentially the same. Management is focused on "maintaining acceptable gas exchange while limiting ventilator associated lung injury,"[24] and pulmonary support includes using ventilator modes that allow spontaneous breathing and cough, using positive end expiratory pressure, and limiting the use of sedation and neuromuscular blocking agents when possible. Prone positioning and extracorporeal membrane oxygenation may be beneficial in more severe cases.[24]

Neurologic

In patients exhibiting neurologic complications, neurologic status should be closely monitored via frequent Glasgow Coma Scale assessments and serial neurologic examinations. Intracranial pressure monitoring may be considered in patients with cerebral edema. Analgesia and sedation should be used judiciously and in conjunction with a sedation/agitation scale to optimize both patient comfort and neurologic examination. neuromuscular blocking agents should be avoided if possible.[24]

Cardiovascular

Intravascular volume should be maintained to limit shock states, because shock may exacerbate lung injury. Albumin has been recommended for volume resuscitation because it binds to fatty acids and, therefore, may decrease the extent of lung injury.[23,24] In patients who develop obstructive shock and right ventricular failure, dobutamine, rather than norepinephrine, may be a more effective agent for hemodynamic support due to its increased inotropic properties. Nitric oxide may also be considered to decrease pulmonary artery pressure and unload the right ventricle.[24]

PREVENTION
Stabilization of Fractures

The incidence of FE and FES in patients with isolated and multiple fractures has been extensively studied over the years; in particular, fractures of the femur have been shown to be a major risk factor.[2,3,6,14,24,25] In addition, other related serious conditions can occur in multiple-injury patients with fractures, including ALI, ARDS, systemic inflammatory response syndrome, and multiple organ dysfunction syndrome.[10] Furthermore, the extent and severity of accompanying injuries may have an impact on the technique and timing of fracture treatment.[10,26,27] Therefore, the optimal approach to treat fractures that minimizes the risk of FES and other serious conditions involves several considerations that present a complex picture that only recently has gained some clarity.[28–31]

For stable patients with only isolated femoral shaft fractures, early internal fixation in less than 10 hours after injury was shown to minimize the risk of FES.[32] In this study, the incidence of FES from a subgroup of 169 patients who were under the age of 35 years was found to be 10.1% for those treated more than 10 hours after injury, but of the 60 patients treated within 10 hours there were no reported incidences of FES.

In patients with multiple injuries and femoral fractures, Bone and colleagues[33] reported a substantial reduction in the incidence of pulmonary complications, including FES and ARDS, with early internal fixation within 24 hours of injury. In this study, 27% percent of the late treatment group (>48 hours) with multiple injuries developed serious respiratory complications compared with 2% of the early treatment group. Riska and Myllynen[34] reported that 22% of the 384 patients treated nonoperatively developed FES in a study specifically dealing with the occurrence of FES in multiple-injury patients with long bone fractures. At the same time, only 4.5% of the 245 patients treated by internal fixation developed clinical FES. This was then followed by a similar group of 211 patients with multiple injuries that was treated with early internal fixation and only 1.4% of this group developed clinical FES.[34] A more recent review by Olson[35] concluded that early definitive treatment of long bone fractures in polytraumatized patients that are hemodynamically stable and appropriately resuscitated led to clear reductions in patient morbidity and mortality.

Blokhuis and colleagues[28] present an alternate view and suggest that timing of definitive fixation may not necessarily play a role in the prevention of FES. Their investigation contends that many of the studies, which evaluated outcomes as related to timing of internal fixation did not specifically take FES into account because the incidence was too low. They conclude that despite advances in treatment strategy for definitive fixation, FES cannot be prevented in all multiple-injury patients but that screening for the symptoms of FES should be done as part of the preoperative work-up prior to the definitive fixation of major fractures. If clinical symptoms of FES or other physiologic instabilities are present, delayed fixation is recommended to avoid additional complications that may be induced by the surgical procedure.

Complexities arise in the evaluation of data that attempts to determine an optimal treatment strategy for FES in multiple-injury patients due to a variety of considerations in past studies. Despite the numerous parameters and potential confounding factors, however, there is general agreement that for patients with multiple injuries, appropriate resuscitation and early fixation of fractures involving long bones is one of the most important treatment strategies to prevent or minimize the severity of FES.[3,10,32–35]

Intraoperative Strategies

FE formation and FES are well-known risk factors associated with major orthopedic procedures, especially those involving the femur. By implementing certain intraoperative techniques that reduce marrow contents and limit intramedullary pressure, however, these risks can be decreased. Christie and colleagues[36] showed that a thorough intramedullary saline lavage prior to cemented hip hemiarthroplasty decreased the duration of embolic response and the number of large emboli compared with minimal lavage. In addition, patients who received the thorough lavage showed less disturbances in end-tidal CO_2 and oxygen saturation, indicating that thorough lavage was also associated with improved pulmonary function.[36]

Pitto and colleagues[37] used a drainage technique during the portion of total hip arthroplasty in which a cemented stem was inserted into the femoral canal. This technique involved suction along the linea aspera to create a vacuum effect in the proximal femoral canal and reduce intramedullary pressure and was shown to significantly lower the occurrence of embolic phenomenon in comparison to conventional stem placement. Patients in the conventional technique group were noted to have signs of cardiopulmonary impairment including a decrease in blood pressure, a decrease in arterial oxygen saturation (Sao_2), and an increase in pulmonary shunt values, which were associated with embolization during stem insertion. In contrast, patients in the drainage technique group only experienced a moderate decrease in Sao_2 and did not show any significant changes in blood pressure or pulmonary shunt values.[37] In a subsequent study, this drainage technique was also correlated with decreased incidence of postoperative deep vein thrombosis.[38]

Corticosteroids

Evidence has suggested that corticosteroids may be effective at preventing FES associated with long bone fractures. A meta-analysis by Bederman and colleagues[39] included 6 trials with a total of 389 patients who had at least 1 long bone fracture. Results revealed that prophylactic corticosteroid administration reduced the risk of FES by 43% to 92% and significantly decreased the risk of hypoxia. In addition, there were no significant differences in mortality and infection associated with corticosteroid administration. It was also shown that lower-dose corticosteroid regimens were more beneficial than those of higher doses.[39] A subsequent literature review by Sen and colleagues[40] showed that only 4% of the 223 patients treated with corticosteroids developed FES compared with 23% of the 260 patients who did not receive corticosteroids.

Despite their apparent efficacy at decreasing the risk of FES, Bederman and colleagues[39] and Sen and colleagues[40] concluded that there is currently insufficient evidence to be able to safely recommend the use of corticosteroids for FES prophylaxis. The investigators expressed concerns about small sample sizes, variable study quality, inconsistent diagnostic criteria for FES, and the large time span during which these studies were conducted due to the major changes that have occurred in the management of trauma and orthopedic injuries. There is also significant concern about the myriad potential adverse effects related to the use of systemic corticosteroids. Further research is required to identify the high-risk patients for whom the benefits of corticosteroid administration outweigh the risks and to determine optimal dosage.[39,40]

Inhaled corticosteroids may be an effective alternative to systemic corticosteroids. One particular inhaled corticosteroid, ciclesonide, has been shown to reach the lung parenchyma unlike most other inhaled corticosteroids. Because it has minimal effect on endogenous cortisol and its systemic absorption is negligible, ciclesonide poses less risk of the adverse effects associated with systemic corticosteroids. Agarwal and colleagues[41] conducted a small study on patients with at least 1 femur fracture, and although their results did not show any statistically significant differences, there was a trend toward decreased incidence of clinical FES and improved oxygenation in the patients who received prophylactic ciclesonide compared with those who did not.

SUMMARY

FES is a potentially lethal complication typically associated with femoral fractures and with orthopedic procedures involving the femur. Currently, the best treatment of FES is prevention and early detection. Early fixation of fractures in appropriate surgical candidates is likely the most effective preventative measure. Corticosteroids, although apparently effective at decreasing risk of FES, require further evaluation by a large randomized trial with definitive diagnostic criteria for FES and standardized dosing regimens before they can be safely recommended for prophylaxis. High-risk patients should be monitored closely for subclinical signs of respiratory insufficiency, and, once FES is suspected, pulmonary, neurologic, and cardiovascular support should be started promptly.

REFERENCES

1. Kosova E, Bergmark B, Piazza G. Fat embolism syndrome. Circulation 2015;131: 317–20.

2. Mellor A, Soni N. Fat embolism. Anaesthesia 2001;56:145–54.
3. Akhtar S. Fat embolism. Anesthesiol Clin 2009;27(3):533–50.
4. George J, George R, Dixit R, et al. Fat embolism syndrome. Lung India 2013; 30(1):47–53.
5. Bulger EM, Smith DG, Maier RV, et al. Fat embolism syndrome. A 10-year review. Arch Surg 1997;132:426–54.
6. Stein PD, Yaekoub AY, Matta F, et al. Fat embolism syndrome. Am J Med Sci 2008;336:472–7.
7. Talbot M, Schemitsch EH. Fat embolism syndrome: history, definition, epidemiology. Injury 2006;37S:S3–7.
8. McAdam L, Rastogi A, Macleod K, et al. Fat embolism syndrome following minor trauma in Duchenne muscular dystrophy. Neuromuscul Disord 2012;22:1035–9.
9. Tsitsikas DA, Gallinella G, Patel S, et al. Bone marrow necrosis and fat embolism syndrome in sickle cell disease: Increased susceptibility of patients with non-SS genotypes and a possible association with human parvovirus B19 infection. Blood Rev 2014;28:23–30.
10. Robinson CM. Current concepts of respiratory insufficiency syndromes after fracture. J Bone Joint Surg Br 2001;83(6):781–91.
11. Rahman SA, Valliani A, Chanda A. Fat embolism syndrome. Fat Embolism Syndrome. Intensive Care 2017. https://doi.org/10.5772/intechopen.69815. InTech.
12. Sulek CA, Davies LK, Enneking FK, et al. Cerebral microembolism diagnosed by transcranial Doppler during total knee arthroplasty: correlation with transesophageal echocardiography. Anesthesiology 1999;91(3):672–6.
13. Nikolic S, Zivkovic V, Babic D, et al. Systemic fat embolism and the patent foramen ovale - A prospective autopsy study. Injury 2012;43:608–12.
14. Johnson MJ, Lucas GL. Fat embolism syndrome. Orthopedics 1996;19(1):41–9.
15. Tzioupis CC, Giannoudis PV. Fat embolism syndrome: what have we learned over the years? Trauma 2011;30(4):259–81.
16. Gurd AR, Wilson RI. The fat embolism syndrome. J Bone Joint Surg Br 1974; 56(3):408–16.
17. Lindeque BG, Schoeman HS, Dommissee GF, et al. Fat embolism and the fat embolism syndrome. A double-blind therapeutic study. J Bone Joint Surg Br 1987; 69(1):123–31.
18. Newbigin K, Souza CA, Torres C, et al. Fat embolism syndrome: state-of-the-art review focused on pulmonary imaging findings. Respir Med 2016;113:93–100.
19. Han YT, Tang J, Gao ZQ, et al. Clinical features and neuroimaging findings in patients with cerebral fat embolism. Chin Med J 2016;129(7):874–6.
20. Koch S, Forteza A, Lavernia C, et al. Cerebral fat microembolism and cognitive decline after hip and knee replacement. Stroke 2007;38(3):1079–81.
21. Barak M, Kabha M, Norman D, et al. Cerebral microemboli during hip fracture fixation: a prospective study. Anesth Analg 2008;107(1):221–5.
22. Riding G, Daly K, Hutchinson S, et al. Paradoxical cerebral fat embolism. An explanation for fat embolism syndrome. J Bone Joint Surg Br 2004;86(1):95–8.
23. Shaikh N. Emergency management of fat embolism syndrome. J Emerg Trauma Shock 2009;2(1):29–33.
24. Habashi NM, Andrews PL, Scalea TM. Therapeutic aspects of fat embolism syndrome. Injury 2006;37S:S68–73.
25. Gossling HR, Pellegrini VD Jr. Fat embolism syndrome: a review of the pathophysiology and physiological basis of treatment. Clin Orthop Relat Res 1982;(165):68–82.

26. O'Toole RV, O'Brien M, Scalea TM, et al. Resuscitation before stabilization of femoral fractures limits acute respiratory distress syndrome in patients with multiple traumatic injuries despite low use of damage control orthopedics. J Trauma 2009;67:1013–21.
27. Pape HC, Rixen D, Morley J, et al. Impact of the method of initial stabilization for femoral shaft fractures in patients with multiple injuries at risk for complications (borderline patients). Ann Surg 2007;246(3):491–9.
28. Blokhuis TJ, Pape H, Frolke J. Timing of definitive fixation of major long bone fractures: Can fat embolism syndrome be prevented? Injury 2017;48S:S3–6.
29. Nahm NJ, Vallier HA. Timing of definitive treatment of femoral shaft fractures in patients with multiple injuries: a systematic review of randomized and non-randomized trials. J Trauma Acute Care Surg 2012;73(5):1046–63.
30. Scalea TM, Boswell SA, Scott JD, et al. External fixation as a bridge to intramedullary nailing for patients with multiple injuries and with femur fractures: damage control orthopedics. J Trauma 2000;48:613–21 [discussion: 621–3].
31. Gandhi RR, Overton TL, Haut ER, et al. Optimal timing of femur fracture stabilization in polytrauma patients: a practice management guideline from the Eastern Association for the Surgery of Trauma. J Trauma Acute Care Surg 2014;77(5):787–95.
32. Pinney SJ, Keating JF, Meek RN. Fat embolism syndrome in isolated femoral fractures: does timing of nailing influence incidence? Injury 1998;29(2):131–3.
33. Bone LB, Johnson KD, Weigel J, et al. Early versus delayed stabilization of femoral fractures: a prospective randomized study. J Bone Joint Surg Am 1989;71(3):336–40.
34. Riska EB, Myllynen P. Fat embolism in patients with multiple injuries. J Trauma 1982;22(11):891–4.
35. Olson SA. Pulmonary aspects of treatment of long bone fractures in the polytrauma patient. Clin Orthop Relat Res 2004;422:66–70.
36. Christie J, Robinson CM, Singer B, et al. Medullary lavage reduces embolic phenomena and cardiopulmonary changes during cemented hip arthroplasty. J Bone Joint Surg Br 1995;77:456–9.
37. Pitto RP, Schramm M, Hohmann D, et al. Relevance of the drainage along the linea aspera for the reduction of fat embolism during cemented total hip arthroplasty. A prospective, randomized clinical trial. Arch Orthop Trauma Surg 1999;199(3–4):146–50.
38. Issack PS, Lauerman MH, Helfet DL, et al. Fat embolism and respiratory distress associated with cemented femoral arthroplasty. Am J Orthop 2009;38(2):72–6.
39. Bederman SS, Bhandari M, McKee MD, et al. Do corticosteroids reduce the risk of fat embolism syndrome in patient with long-bone fractures? A meta-analysis. Can J Surg 2009;52(5):386–93.
40. Sen RK, Tripathy SK, Krishnan V. Role of corticosteroids as a prophylactic measure in fat embolism syndrome: a literature review. Musculoskelet Surg 2012;96:1–8.
41. Agarwal AK, Sen R, Tripathy SK, et al. Is there any role of inhalational corticosteroids in the prophylaxis of post-traumatic fat embolism syndrome? Cureus 2015;7(9):e332.

Diagnosis and Treatment of Common Pain Syndromes and Disorders

Brett Morgan, DNP, CRNA[a],*, Steve Wooden, DNP, CRNA, NSPM[b]

KEYWORDS

- Pain syndromes • Chronic pain • Diagnosis • Treatment • Primary care

KEY POINTS

- As more patients access the health care system for the management of pain-related disorders, providers will be challenged with seeking appropriate methods of treatment.
- It is essential for all care givers to have a general understanding of common pain syndromes, and how to appropriately manage the care of patients with chronic pain.
- A pain specialist will continue to provide care and expertise for complex patients; however, limitations in access to comprehensive pain care will necessitate the use of primary care for a large portion of pain-related health care.

INTRODUCTION

The management of patients with chronic pain has become a significant challenge for primary care providers. It is projected that as many as 1 out of every 10 Americans will develop chronic pain at some point over their life course, and the cost is staggering. Recent estimates suggest that the treatment of pain-related syndrome in the United States costs as much as $635 billion a year.[1]

Although some patients receive treatment for pain in specialty pain clinics, the majority will access care in a primary setting. Because chronic pain is widespread and increasing, most health care providers will see patients with chronic or severe pain resulting from any number of disease states. Treatment protocols for patients in pain requires specialized knowledge of the pain's etiology and evidence-based approaches to manage the pain. The goal of this review is to provide an overview of common pain syndromes seen in the primary care setting and to highlight current treatment options for those syndromes.

Disclosure Statement: Neither author has any commercial or financial conflicts to disclose related to this article.
[a] Duke University School of Nursing, Nurse Anesthesia Program, 307 Trent Drive, Durham, NC 27710, USA; [b] Department of Anesthesia, Wooden Anesthesia PC, Boone County Medical Center, 406 S 8th Street, Albion, NE 68620, USA
* Corresponding author.
E-mail address: Brett.morgan@duke.edu

Nurs Clin N Am 53 (2018) 349–360
https://doi.org/10.1016/j.cnur.2018.04.004
0029-6465/18/Published by Elsevier Inc.
nursing.theclinics.com

MYOFASCIAL PAIN SYNDROME

Myofascial pain syndrome (MFP) is a noninflammatory disorder of the musculoskeletal system associated with pain and stiffness. It is thought to be caused by repetitive injury to the muscles, but can occur with a single injury. Contributing factors include autoimmune dysfunction, connective tissue disorders such as lupus and rheumatoid arthritis, stress, and depression. Patients present with musculoskeletal pain, limited mobility, weakness, and referred pain. MFP can begin at any age, but is most commonly seen in women ages 15 to 40. Estrogen seems to play a significant role in the development of MFP.[2]

The most significant physical finding in MFP is the presence of hyperirritable palpable nodules in the skeletal muscle fibers referred to as myofascial trigger points.[3] Fibromyalgia (FM) and MFP are often confused with each other because symptomatology often overlaps. Individuals with either of these disorders may exhibit headaches, abdominal and pelvic pain, dysmenorrhea, prostatitis, and irritable bowel. The distinct, but difficult to ascertain difference, is that FM is centrally mediated and MFP is a peripheral disorder in which pain originates within the muscle at myofascial trigger points.[4]

Diagnosis

The most significant finding in a patient with MFP is a tight band within a muscle group that has a reproducible localized point of tenderness. The pain duration should be greater than 3 months, and the patient should not have another disorder that would account for the pain. The initial evaluation of a patient suspected with MFP is very important. Positive findings should include areas of pain that can be reproduced by provocative maneuvers. They should be consistent and not wandering. In addition, the identified point of most intense pain should produce referred pain along the muscle when stimulated for a few seconds.[5] The primary clinical finding in MFP is referred pain. The patterns of referral often do not make neurologic sense. For example, pain from a trigger point in the trapezius, innervated by cranial nerve XI, may refer to the forehead, innervated by cranial nerve V. However, the clinical presentation, characteristic referral, and the response to local anesthetic or other peripheral treatments are accepted by most providers to meet diagnostic criteria.[6]

Treatment

Pharmacologic treatment, typically used to combat most pain syndromes, includes nonsteroidal antiinflammatory drugs (NSAIDs). However, beyond the analgesic properties of NSAIDS, it is likely that they are not helpful because the syndrome is noninflammatory. Muscle relaxants, such as tizanidine, have been shown to support significant improvement in pain intensity. Benzodiazepines also decrease pain symptoms in MFP through inhibition of neurotransmission. Anticonvulsants such as gabapentin and pregabalin have been used to treat MFP, but there is little evidence of their effectiveness. The use of Duloxetine, a serotonin-norepinephrine reuptake inhibitor, has been shown to be a useful adjunct to improve mood and treatment compliance, although little evidence exists to suggest the use of other classes of antidepressants for the treatment of MFP.[7]

Some interventional therapies have shown promise in the treatment of MFP. Deactivating the myofascial trigger point is essential in treatment. Cryotherapy, muscles stretching, ultrasound therapy, dry needling, and local anesthetic injections have been used with varying degrees of success. Cryotherapy, or cold compression therapy, is controversial among providers. Some feel that cold therapy inhibits hyperactive neurotransmission, whereas others feel that cold therapy aggravates the symptoms. There are no good studies that demonstrate the effectiveness of cold therapy[8] or the regular use of ultrasound therapy.[9] Other controversial procedures include injection of botulinum toxin into the myofascial trigger point, aggressive physical therapy, and periodic injections of local anesthetic. Studies have yet to demonstrate the long-term effectiveness of any of these methods.

Dry needling is a therapeutic treatment that is thought to reduce muscle hyperexcitability, break up scar tissue, and improve circulation to the myofascial trigger point. Therapeutic needling is performed with sterile 32-G, 80-mm acupuncture needles. A small needle is first used to pierce the skin and muscle, and serves to identify the appropriate location for placement of the acupuncture needle. The smaller needle is removed, and the acupuncture needle is inserted further into the taut band to elicit a twitch response. Appropriate placement of the needle is confirmed by reproduction of recognizable pain or by observation of local twitch response. The needle is then partially withdrawn and repeatedly inserted into the muscle until no further twitches are observed. After inactivating trigger points and reducing referred pain, passive stretching is performed, which lengthens the muscle to its normal state. Stretching in combination with dry needling provides the most effective outcome. Patients typically receive 8 needling protocols administered over an 8-week period[10] and patients are asked to continue stretching. Long-term relief from MFP symptoms using dry needling seems possible.

FIBROMYALGIA

FM is a centrally mediated syndrome characterized by chronic widespread pain, fatigue, and psychological symptoms such as depression and anxiety. In addition, patients often experience an increased sensitivity to touch (ie, tender points) with the absence of systemic or localized inflammation.[11] It can be a severely debilitating disorder and affects an estimated 1 in 20 individuals in the United States,[12] and is most common in women at a ratio of 9:1. It can occur in all races, ethnicities, socioeconomic classes, and age groups.[13] Unlike MFP, which is a peripherally mediated dysfunction, FM arises from the central nervous system. Although the cause is unclear, there is increasing evidence that genetic factors may play an important role in the development of FM, particularly alterations in genes that affect stress response neurotransmitters, such as serotonin and dopamine, along with catecholamines. Most practitioners believe that FM is not an autoimmune, inflammatory, or muscle disorder, but that it accompanies inflammatory conditions such as osteoarthritis, lupus, and rheumatoid arthritis, and should be considered as a comorbid condition with those diseases.[11,12]

Diagnosis

FM is characterized by a set of unique clinical signs and symptoms that lends it to diagnosis by primary care providers. Studies have shown that patients who receive a formal diagnosis of FM respond better to treatment, use health care resources less, and report a greater satisfaction with their care. A detailed history and physical examination is an important initial step in the diagnosis of FM.[12] The diagnosis should be considered when patients report diffuse or multifocal pain, and that consideration should increase if patients demonstrate progression of that pain over multiple visits. Because conditions such as hypothyroidism, rheumatoid arthritis, osteoarthritis, adrenal dysfunction, and multiple myeloma are conditions that may mimic FM, they should be ruled out before a final diagnosis is made. In addition, psychiatric diagnoses, such as posttraumatic stress disorder, anxiety disorders, and depression may account for symptoms similar to FM. If a patient exhibiting symptoms of FM is found to have a newly diagnosed mental health disorder, treating the mental health disorder might alleviate the problem altogether.[14]

In 2010, the American College of Rheumatology developed a clear set of diagnostic criteria for FM. Their recommendations include the administration of a Wide Spread Pain Index (WPI) and Symptom Severity Inventory (SSI). The WPI assesses the number of areas in which a patient has experiences pain during the previous 6 months. The areas are divides into 6 lower extremity, 6 upper extremity, and 7 axial skeletal locations. A final score is calculated between 0 and 19. The SSI calculates the sum of severity of general somatic symptoms, waking unrefreshed cognitive symptoms, and severity of fatigue. Each of the symptoms are assessed on a scale of 0 to 3, where 0 is no pain and 3 is severe pain. The final score is calculated between 0 and 12. The American College of Rheumatology diagnostic criteria for FM are[11,12]:

- WPI of 7 or greater and an SSI of 5 or greater; or
- WPI of 3 to 6 and SSI of 9 or greater; and
- Symptoms have been present as for greater than 3 months and the patient does not have a disorder that would otherwise explain the pain.

Treatment

Several treatments have been used for patients with FM, with varying rates of success. Pharmacologic treatments include antidepressants, antiseizure medications, judicious use of muscle relaxants. A metaanalysis of more than 5000 patients with FM who took 2 or more of these classes of drugs indicated a 30% pain reduction over those patients on a placebo.[15] Although pharmacologic treatments are preferred by patients and providers because of their convenience and simplicity, there are a number of nonpharmacologic treatments that show promise for long-term success in the treatment of FM. Exercise therapy, acupuncture, psychiatric therapy, cognitive-behavioral therapy, and biofeedback demonstrate effectiveness, especially when customized to suit the individual patient to ensure effectiveness and compliance. Common treatments for FM along with recommendations for initiation are found in **Table 1**.[11,12]

CHRONIC POSTSURGICAL PAIN

Chronic postsurgical pain (CPSP) is a particularly troublesome type of chronic pain that occurs after as many as one-half of surgeries.[16] A clear definition and reasons for this syndrome are difficult to pin down.[17] Although the pain seems to be neuropathic in nature, it is not always associated with identifiable nerve injury.[18,19] The International Association for the Study of Pain defines CPSP as persistent pain more than 2 months after a surgery that cannot be explained by recurrence of disease, apparent inflammation, or other reason.

Research into CPSP has identified a group of the most common surgical procedures associated with the syndrome and potential methods to predict and prevent its occurrence. Surgical procedures associated with CPSP include mastectomy, thoracotomy, cholecystectomy, nephrectomy, sternotomy, and other chest and upper abdominal procedures. Other common types of surgery that report a high incidence of CPSP are amputation and inguinal/pelvic surgical procedures such as hernia repair. Nearly 1 in 4 patients who undergo thoracic surgery develop CPSP, but only one-third of them have an identifiable nerve injury.[20] This finding suggests that multiple factors are responsible for CPSP.

Table 1
Treatments for fibromyalgia

Treatment	Recommendation
Pharmacologic	
Pregabalin (gabapentinoid)	300–400 mg/d Start at 75 mg twice a day Gradually increase to a maximum dose of 225 mg twice a day
Duloxetine (serotonin-norepinephrine reuptake inhibitor)	60 mg/d; starting 30 mg/d then increasing after 1 wk
Milnacipran (serotonin-norepinephrine reuptake inhibitor)	100 mg/d (maximum dose), start at 12.5 mg and increase incrementally to the maximum dose
Nonpharmacologic	
Exercise	To improve physical function, begin slowly with low-impact activity and increase to moderate activity over time
Cognitive-behavioral therapy	Use face-to-face counseling, online resources, and reading materials to provide knowledge about fibromyalgia, and potential coping strategies
Complementary and alternative medical therapies	Consider recommending yoga, acupuncture, massage, or alternative diets to improve pain control and overall function

Diagnosis

Predictors of CPSP help to isolate likely candidates, but do little to identify a treatable source of pain. The existence of preoperative pain, either functional or psychological, seems to be a predictor of CPSP. In at least 1 study, preoperative pain was the most significant clinical predictor of CPSP.[21] However, other studies indicate multiple predictive factors, such as thyroid function, occult wound infection, or even secondary gain as contributors to CPSP.[22] There are few factors that predict a lower incidence of CPSP, such as younger patient age and immunosuppressant therapy.[23] The latter suggests that patients who are immunosuppressed postoperatively have a significantly lower incidence of CPSP when compared with those who are not.

Treatment

Treating CPSP can be challenging. Research has pointed to the benefits of preventative measures that reduce central sensitization, which can be accomplished by using regional anesthesia, giving preoperative doses of antiinflammatory agents, and administering other antihyperalgesia medications such as ketamine.[24–26]

Treatment goals for CPSP should be multifaceted and begin with removal of the stimulus, typically at or near the surgical site. Then, it is important to reset the inhibitory mechanisms of the central spinal area and address the psychological impact of chronic pain.

Aggressive postoperative treatment seems to be important in the treatment of CPSP. Some pharmaceuticals are effective in reducing the dysfunctional activity associated with the syndrome, some are effective in helping the body return to normal function, and others simply treat pain perception. Tricyclic antidepressants have been shown to be useful in treating CPSP, in addition to the short-term use of opioids such as morphine use and selective use of anticonvulsants, topical agents, and N-methyl-D-aspartate receptor (NMDA) antagonists.[27]

Finding solutions to CPSP can be very elusive. That is why preventative measures are important. Research has pointed to the benefits of preventative measures that reduce central sensitization. This can be accomplished using regional anesthesia, preoperative doses of antiinflammatory agents, and administration of other antihyperalgesia medications such as ketamine.

NSAIDs can be used to mitigate the development of CPSP and treat ongoing pain. Drugs in this category have antipyretic, antiinflammatory, and analgesic properties. Although acetaminophen is often included in this category, it is not a true NSAID because it lacks significant antiinflammatory properties. Acetaminophen does have inhibitory cyclooxygenase activity, but it is thought to provide this inhibition in the central nervous system rather than peripherally. This agent provides pain relief through a decrease in nociceptor activity in the central nervous system.[28]

Like acetaminophen, opioids act primarily on the central nervous system. This property prevents them from being useful in treating the source of pain, but they are valuable for short-term relief of postoperative pain, traumatic injury, and CPSP. Opioid therapy for CPSP is not a good long-term solution because of the substantial negative side effects, including physical dependence and increased risk of opioid overdose. In addition to potentially fatal side effects, tolerance develops over time, which decreases the therapeutic value and increases risks associated with addiction and depression.[29]

Antidepressants should be considered as a first-line treatment for CPSP[30] because pain perception is a chemically mediated event in the central nervous system. Antidepressants can improve mood, increase treatment compliance, and decrease opioid use. These medications can take weeks to be effective, so they are not appropriate for acute postoperative pain, nor do they seem to be an effective CPSP preventative strategy. Extended-release compounds seem to be most effective in the treatment of CPSP. Side effects are generally well-tolerated. Antidepressants are sometimes rejected by patients as a treatment for chronic pain because they may feel that taking this class of drugs will label them as psychologically impaired. It is important to explain to patients that some drugs designed for 1 purpose are beneficial for other purposes. Anticonvulsants are one such drug. Their use for chronic neuropathic pain, including CPSP, is controversial. Some studies have found little to no value in using anticonvulsants for chronic neuropathic pain, whereas others have demonstrated efficacy for specific anticonvulsants such as gabapentin and pregabalin.[31,32]

It is thought that NMDA receptor systems are involved in the development of chronic pain wind-up, and preemptive treatment may be effective in the prevention of postoperative pain hypersensitivity. NMDA receptors are thought to support synaptic plasticity, central nervous system pain processing, and modulation of central pain sensitization induced by incision and tissue damage,[33] which may suggest their value in the treatment and prevention of CPSP. Ketamine, for example, blocks NMDA receptor site activity.

Topical anesthetic agents are effective with CPSP because some chronic pain conditions continually stimulate peripheral nerves. Topical NSAIDs and anesthetic agents have a high therapeutic benefit and are safer than ingested medications when used in therapeutic doses.[34] Although side effects, most commonly skin irritation, are mild, topicals remain an underused tool in the battle against chronic pain and CPSP probably owing to the relative costs. Application of anesthetic agents to the source of pain may promote reestablishment of the normal peripheral nociceptive inhibitory systems by temporarily blocking continuous nerve stimulation.

Treatment of CPSP is far more complex than simply addressing a single source of pain. The syndrome includes a cycle of dysfunction that leads to a breakdown in homeostasis. Return to homeostasis requires addressing peripheral, spinal, and cerebral mechanisms that have broken down owing to repetitive painful stimulation. It is important to identify patients who might be predisposed to CPSP, use preemptive treatments, diagnose CPSP quickly, and aggressively treat the condition. The longer treatment is delayed, the more likely the problem will become irreversible or unmanageable.

COMPLEX REGIONAL PAIN SYNDROME

Complex regional pain syndrome (CRPS) describes a variety of chronic pain conditions associated with persistent pain that is out of proportion with any associated tissue injury.[35,36] Although it is not restricted to any particular anatomic region of the body, CRPS usually begins in the distal extremities and is distinguished by the presence of autonomic and inflammatory changes in the region of an associated injury. It is estimated to effect as many as 26 of every 100,000 persons annually.[37]

CRPS can be subdivided into 2 categories. Type I CRPS describes a condition that is associated with a recognized peripheral nerve injury, whereas type II CRPS has no identified injury.[35] For many years, it was assumed that the sympathetic nervous system plays an important role in the development of CRPS. In fact, until recently, the name associated with the syndrome was reflex sympathetic dystrophy.[38] This was due to a common clinical presentation of cold and sweaty affected extremities. Because CRPS presents in a diverse manner, it is now believed that multiple mechanisms are responsible for the development of the syndrome. The most commonly accepted potential mechanisms involved in the development of CRPS are listed in **Box 1**. CRPS can be further classified as either being acute in nature or chronic. Acute CRPS is defined as symptomatic disease for less than 1 year and chronic (ie, symptoms for >1 year).[36]

Diagnosis

CRPS is a diagnosis of exclusion. The lack of a directly understood pathophysiologic mechanism for CRPS supports the use of objective medical testing as a method for ruling out other conditions. Because the exact mechanism associated with the development of CRPS is not understood, the diagnosis is based exclusively on clinical signs and symptoms. First in 1994 and again in 2012, the International Association for the Study of Pain published a consensus guideline for the diagnosis of CRPS. The most recent guidelines require both subjective symptoms and objective signs gathered by physical examination.[39] Current diagnostic criteria for CRPS are presented in **Box 2**.

Treatment

Studies suggest that most cases of acute CRPS will resolve with conservative medical treatment. However, chronic CRPS often requires a multidisciplinary approach,

---

Box 1
Commonly accepted mechanisms of the development of complex regional pain syndrome

- Initial and direct nerve injury.[41,44]
- Reperfusion injuries after ischemia.[41,45]
- Structural and function changes to the brain after injury.[46–48]
- Central and peripheral sensitization after tissue injury.[41]
- Psychological factors such as depression and anxiety in conjunction with physical distress.[41]

Box 2
International Association for the Study of Pain diagnostic criteria for complex regional pain syndrome

- Continuous pain that is disproportionate to the precipitating injury
- Report 1 symptom in 3 of the 4 following categories:
  - Sensory: Patient reports allodynia or hyperalgesia;
  - Vasomotor: Patient reports skin color changes, changes in color symmetry, or temperature asymmetry;
  - Sudomotor/edema: Patient describes edema, sweating changes, and or sweating asymmetry; or
  - Motor/trophic: Decreased range of motion, motor dysfunction, and or trophic changes.
- Physical assessment reveals evidence of 1 sign in 2 or more of the following:
  - Sensory: Allodynia to light touch, joint movement, or deep somatic pressure, and/or hyperalgesia to a pinprick;
  - Vasomotor: Skin temperature asymmetry, and or skin color changes/asymmetry;
  - Sudomotor: Edema, sweating changes, and or sweating asymmetry; and
  - Motor/trophic: Decreased range of motion, motor dysfunction, and or trophic changes.
- There is no other diagnosis that better explains the patients signs or symptoms.

---

including pharmacologic approaches, psychological treatment and therapy, and physical and occupational therapy. Owing to the need for higher quality clinical trials for the treatment of CRPS, most treatments lack research validation. Thus, treatment often relies on the clinical judgment pain experts, who should be called to consult in the care of these patients.[36] Common approaches to the treatment of CRPS are:

- Corticosteroid treatment (often the first-line pharmacologic treatment)[40];
- Gabapentin and other anticonvulsants[41];
- Sympathetic ganglion blocks (stellate ganglion, lumbar sympathetic)[42];
- Spinal cord stimulation[43]; and
- Cognitive-behavioral therapy.[36]

PAINFUL DIABETIC NEUROPATHY

Painful diabetic neuropathy (PDN) is a common condition found in patients with type 1 and type 2 diabetes. It is characterized by diffuse damage to peripheral nerve fibers, which results in multiple neuropathic symptoms, including pain, numbness, and paresthesia.[44] Up to 90% of patients with diabetes report some degree of peripheral neuropathy, and up to 34% of those patients report some degree of pain associated with those symptoms.[45,46]

Unlike nonpainful diabetic neuropathy, PDN is associated with a significant decrease in quality of life. Patients with PDN describe symptoms of burning, stabbing, and electrical pain, along with hyperalgesia and severe pain with innocuous stimuli. In addition, patients report significant and debilitating sleep deprivation, depression, anxiety, and limitations to physical function.[44] Considering that up to 39% of patients with PDN go untreated, there is potential for a significant impact on health care systems, and this will likely increase as the epidemic of diabetes grows.[47]

Diagnosis

PDN is diagnosed primarily using clinical findings found during a thorough patient history and physical examination. For patients with diabetes who also experience numbness, it is likely unnecessary to confirm neuropathy using diagnostic testing to check for large nerve fiber deficits. Instead, patient assessment should focus on gathering a comprehensive description of the patient's pain. Common descriptives may include:

- Continuous or intermittent,
- Symmetric or distributed,
- Burning, stabbing, or tingling,
- Hot or cold, and
- Heightened or reduced perceptions of temperature or touch.

In addition to subjective patient interviews, the severity of PDN can be assessed using pain scores derived from assessments such as the Brief Pain Inventory and the Neuropathic Pain Questionnaire. Although these instruments may be helpful in describing the severity of the pain, they have been shown to be less helpful in demonstrating change associated with treatment.[44]

Treatment

After a diagnosis of PDN has been made, treatment can take 1 of 2 courses. The provider can treat the underlying cause of the neuropathy or manage the symptoms associated with PDN.[44] Treating, managing, and preventing hyperglycemia has been shown to prevent further development of diabetic neuropathies and, in some cases, stop or reverse the progression of PDN. Strategies include tight glycemic control with intensive insulin treatment, dietary control, and pharmacologic strategies to improve glucose use and control in type 2 diabetics. Pancreas transplantation has also been shown to reverse diabetic neuropathy and associated syndromes.[44,48]

Symptom management provides a significant challenge to practitioners treating patients with PDN. Numerous clinical guidelines have been released for symptom treatment of patients with PDN; however, consensus among them suggest the use of tricyclic agents, GABA analogues, and serotonin-norepinephrine reuptake inhibitors. In addition, topical treatments have been shown to provide some relief **(Table 2)**.[44,46]

Table 2 First-line treatments for diabetic painful neuropathy	
Drug	**Mechanism of Action**
Tricyclic antidepressant (amitriptyline, imipramine, desipramine)	Inhibit reuptake of noradrenaline and serotonin
GABA analogues (gabapentin, pregabalin)	Reduction of neurotransmitter release by binding to voltage-gated calcium channels
Serotonin-norepinephrine reuptake inhibitors (duloxetine, venlafaxine)	Inhibition of noradrenaline and serotonin reuptake, leading to augmentation of descending inhibitory pathways
Topical creams (capsaicin 0.075%)	Substance P depletion from primary afferent neurons; leads to loss of intraepidermal nerve fiber density

Data from Javed S, Petropoulos IN, Alam U, et al. Treatment of painful diabetic neuropathy. Ther Adv Chronic Dis 2015;6(1):15–28; and Peltier A, Goutman SA, Callaghan BC. Painful diabetic neuropathy. BMJ 2014;348:g1799.

SUMMARY

As more patients access the health care system for management of pain-related disorders, providers will be challenged with seeking appropriate methods of treatment. It is essential for all care givers to have a general understanding of common pain syndromes, and how to appropriately manage the care of patients with chronic pain. A pain specialist will continue to provide care and expertise for complex patients; however, limitations in access to comprehensive pain care will necessitate the use of primary care for a large portion of pain-related health care.

REFERENCES

1. Elder N, Penm M, Pallerla H, et al. Provision of recommended chronic pain assessment and management in primary care: does patient-centered medical home (PCMH) recognition make a difference? J Am Board Fam Med 2016; 29(4):474–81.
2. Hongxing L, Astrom AN, List T, et al. Prevalence of temporomandibular disorder pain in Chinese adolescents compared to an age-matched Swedish population. J Oral Rehabil 2016;43(4):241–8.
3. Saxena A, Chansoria M, Tomar G, et al. Myofascial pain syndrome: an overview. J Pain Palliat Care Pharmacother 2015;29(1):16–21.
4. Ge HY, Wang Y, Fernandez-de-las-Penas C, et al. Reproduction of overall spontaneous pain pattern by manual stimulation of active myofascial trigger points in fibromyalgia patients. Arthritis Res Ther 2011;13(2):R48.
5. Gerwin RD. Diagnosing fibromyalgia and myofascial pain syndrome: a guide. J Fam Pract 2013;62(12 Suppl 1):S19–25.
6. Mense S. The pathogenesis of muscle pain. Curr Pain Headache Rep 2003;7(6): 419–25.
7. Desai MJ, Saini V, Saini S. Myofascial pain syndrome: a treatment review. Pain Ther 2013;2(1):21–36.
8. Ernst E, Fialka V. Ice freezes pain? A review of the clinical effectiveness of analgesic cold therapy. J Pain Symptom Manage 1994;9(1):56–9.
9. van der Windt DA, van der Heijden GJ, van den Berg SG, et al. Ultrasound therapy for musculoskeletal disorders: a systematic review. Pain 1999;81(3):257–71.
10. Huang YT, Lin SY, Neoh CA, et al. Dry needling for myofascial pain: prognostic factors. J Altern Complement Med 2011;17(8):755–62.
11. Hopkins L, Smallheer B. Alterations of musculoskeletal function. In: McCance KL, Huether SE, editors. Pathophysiology: the biologic basis for disease in adults and children. St Louis (MO): Elsevier; 2019. p. 1423–71.
12. Arnold LM, Gebke KB, Choy EH. Fibromyalgia: management strategies for primary care providers. Int J Clin Pract 2016;70(2):99–112.
13. Balkarli A, Erol MK, Yucel O, et al. Frequency of fibromyalgia syndrome in patients with central serous chorioretinopathy. Arq Bras Oftalmol 2017;80(1):4–8.
14. Schneider MJ, Brady DM, Perle SM. Commentary: differential diagnosis of fibromyalgia syndrome: proposal of a model and algorithm for patients presenting with the primary symptom of chronic widespread pain. J Manipulative Physiol Ther 2006;29(6):493–501.
15. Lee YH, Song GG. Comparative efficacy and tolerability of duloxetine, pregabalin, and milnacipran for the treatment of fibromyalgia: a Bayesian network meta-analysis of randomized controlled trials. Rheumatol Int 2016;36(5):663–72.
16. Kehlet H, Rathmell JP. Persistent postsurgical pain: the path forward through better design of clinical studies. Anesthesiology 2010;112(3):514–5.

17. Cregg R, Anwar S, Farquhar-Smith P. Persistent postsurgical pain. Curr Opin Support Palliat Care 2013;7(2):144–52.
18. Steegers MA, Snik DM, Verhagen AF, et al. Only half of the chronic pain after thoracic surgery shows a neuropathic component. J Pain 2008;9(10):955–61.
19. Johansen A, Schirmer H, Nielsen CS, et al. Persistent post-surgical pain and signs of nerve injury: the Tromso Study. Acta Anaesthesiol Scand 2016;60(3):380–92.
20. Peng Z, Li H, Zhang C, et al. A retrospective study of chronic post-surgical pain following thoracic surgery: prevalence, risk factors, incidence of neuropathic component, and impact on quality of life. PLoS One 2014;9(2):e90014.
21. Pinto PR, McIntyre T, Ferrero R, et al. Risk factors for moderate and severe persistent pain in patients undergoing total knee and hip arthroplasty: a prospective predictive study. PLoS One 2013;8(9):e73917.
22. Costa MA, Trentini CA, Schafranski MD, et al. Factors associated with the development of chronic post-sternotomy pain: a case-control study. Braz J Cardiovasc Surg 2015;30(5):552–6.
23. Kristensen AD, Pedersen TA, Hjortdal VE, et al. Chronic pain in adults after thoracotomy in childhood or youth. Br J Anaesth 2010;104(1):75–9.
24. Andreae MH, Andreae DA. Local anaesthetics and regional anaesthesia for preventing chronic pain after surgery. Cochrane Database Syst Rev 2012;(10):CD007105.
25. Lavand'homme P, De Kock M. The use of intraoperative epidural or spinal analgesia modulates postoperative hyperalgesia and reduces residual pain after major abdominal surgery. Acta Anaesthesiol Belg 2006;57(4):373–9.
26. Lavand'homme P, De Kock M, Waterloos H. Intraoperative epidural analgesia combined with ketamine provides effective preventive analgesia in patients undergoing major digestive surgery. Anesthesiology 2005;103(4):813–20.
27. Chaparro LE, Wiffen PJ, Moore RA, et al. Combination pharmacotherapy for the treatment of neuropathic pain in adults. Cochrane Database Syst Rev 2012;(7):CD008943.
28. Hinz B, Cheremina O, Brune K. Acetaminophen (paracetamol) is a selective cyclooxygenase-2 inhibitor in man. FASEB J 2008;22(2):383–90.
29. Volkow ND, McLellan AT. Opioid abuse in chronic pain–misconceptions and mitigation strategies. N Engl J Med 2016;374(13):1253–63.
30. O'Connor AB, Dworkin RH. Treatment of neuropathic pain: an overview of recent guidelines. Am J Med 2009;122(10 Suppl):S22–32.
31. Goodyear-Smith F, Halliwell J. Anticonvulsants for neuropathic pain: gaps in the evidence. Clin J Pain 2009;25(6):528–36.
32. Wiffen P, Collins S, McQuay H, et al. Anticonvulsant drugs for acute and chronic pain. Cochrane Database Syst Rev 2005;(3):CD001133.
33. De Kock MF, Lavand'homme PM. The clinical role of NMDA receptor antagonists for the treatment of postoperative pain. Best Pract Res Clin Anaesthesiol 2007;21(1):85–98.
34. Roth SH, Fuller P. Diclofenac topical solution compared with oral diclofenac: a pooled safety analysis. J Pain Res 2011;4:159–67.
35. Miller C, Williams M, Heine P, et al. Current practice in the rehabilitation of complex regional pain syndrome: a survey of practitioners. Disabil Rehabil 2017;73(2):1–7.
36. Bruehl S. Complex regional pain syndrome. BMJ 2015;351:h2730.
37. de Mos M, de Bruijn AG, Huygen FJ, et al. The incidence of complex regional pain syndrome: a population-based study. Pain 2007;129(1–2):12–20.

38. Schurmann M, Gradl G, Zaspel J, et al. Peripheral sympathetic function as a predictor of complex regional pain syndrome type I (CRPS I) in patients with radial fracture. Auton Neurosci 2000;86(1–2):127–34.

39. International Association for the Study of Pain. Classification of chronic pain. 2nd edition (revised). Seattle (WA): IASP Press; 2017.

40. Atalay NS, Ercidogan O, Akkaya N, et al. Prednisolone in complex regional pain syndrome. Pain Physician 2014;17(2):179–85.

41. van de Vusse AC, Stomp-van den Berg SG, Kessels AH, et al. Randomised controlled trial of gabapentin in Complex Regional Pain Syndrome type 1 [ISRCTN84121379]. BMC Neurol 2004;4:13.

42. O'Connell NE, Wand BM, McAuley J, et al. Interventions for treating pain and disability in adults with complex regional pain syndrome. Cochrane Database Syst Rev 2013;(4):CD009416.

43. Kemler MA, de Vet HC, Barendse GA, et al. Effect of spinal cord stimulation for chronic complex regional pain syndrome type I: five-year final follow-up of patients in a randomized controlled trial. J Neurosurg 2008;108(2):292–8.

44. Javed S, Petropoulos IN, Alam U, et al. Treatment of painful diabetic neuropathy. Ther Adv Chronic Dis 2015;6(1):15–28.

45. Ziegler D, Rathmann W, Dickhaus T, et al. Neuropathic pain in diabetes, prediabetes and normal glucose tolerance: the MONICA/KORA Augsburg Surveys S2 and S3. Pain Med 2009;10(2):393–400.

46. Peltier A, Goutman SA, Callaghan BC. Painful diabetic neuropathy. BMJ 2014; 348:g1799.

47. Daousi C, MacFarlane IA, Woodward A, et al. Chronic painful peripheral neuropathy in an urban community: a controlled comparison of people with and without diabetes. Diabet Med 2004;21(9):976–82.

48. Callaghan BC, Hur J, Feldman EL. Diabetic neuropathy: one disease or two? Curr Opin Neurol 2012;25(5):536–41.

Malabsorption Syndromes

Ricketta Clark, DNP, FNP-BC[a],*, Ragan Johnson, DNP, FNP-BC[b]

KEYWORDS

- Malabsorption • Digestion • Celiac disease • Short bowel syndrome • Maldigestion

KEY POINTS

- Several conditions of the small bowel can be responsible for malabsorption syndromes.
- Understanding multiple diagnostic modalities prevents delayed diagnoses.
- Adequate and early treatment positively affects prognosis.

BACKGROUND

The gastrointestinal (GI) system is responsible for the motility, secretion, regulation, and digestion of nutrients consumed in the diet. Vital to maintaining adequate health is the GI system's multifaceted and complex ability to digest and absorb fluids, electrolytes, macronutrients, and micronutrients.[1] Normal nutrient absorption requires 3 steps[2,3]:

- Luminal and brush border processing
- Absorption into the intestinal mucosa
- Transport into the circulation.

An impairment in intestinal absorption and functioning is known as intestinal insufficiency or deficiency. The European Society for Clinical Nutrition and Metabolism defines intestinal insufficiency or deficiency as a decrease in gut absorptive function not requiring intravenous supplementation for health and/or growth maintenance.[4,5] Malabsorption is impaired absorption of nutrients caused by any disruption in the process of normal absorption. Impaired digestion of nutrients within the intestinal lumen or at the brush border membrane can also interfere with nutrient absorption. This is known as maldigestion. Malabsorption and maldigestion differ pathophysiologically (**Table 1**) but the processes of digestion and absorption are interdependent. Therefore, in clinical practice, malabsorption refers to deficiencies in the process of both absorption and digestion.[3,6]

Disclosure Statement: The authors have nothing to disclose.
[a] Nursing, University of Tennessee Health Science Center, 920 Madison Avenue, Memphis, TN 38163, USA; [b] Nursing, Duke University School of Nursing, 307 Trent Drive, DUMC 3322, Durham, NC 27710, USA
* Corresponding author.
E-mail address: rclark25@uthsc.edu

Nurs Clin N Am 53 (2018) 361–374
https://doi.org/10.1016/j.cnur.2018.05.001
0029-6465/18/© 2018 Elsevier Inc. All rights reserved.

nursing.theclinics.com

| Table 1 |
| Examples of maldigestion and malabsorption |

	Malabsorption	Maldigestion
Etiologic factors	Impaired absorption of digested food caused by alterations of intestinal mucosa	Impaired breakdown of food in intestinal lumen
Examples	Crohn disease Celiac disease Lactose intolerance Small intestine resection Small intestinal bacterial overgrowth Whipple disease Radiation enteritis Pernicious anemia	Pancreatic insufficiency Gastric resection (bariatric) Bile acid deficiency Cirrhosis

Although malabsorption disorders can originate from the liver, pancreas, stomach, or intestines, this article reviews common disorders of the small bowel that result in malabsorption.

ETIOLOGIC FACTORS

Malabsorption can result from congenital defects in the membrane transport system of the small intestine epithelium, from acquired defects, or from surgery.[7] A defect in any of the 3 phases of normal absorption can result in malabsorption, and these defects may exist concurrently.[3] Malabsorption may be either global or partial (isolated). Global malabsorption results from diseases with diffuse small bowel mucosal involvement or reduced absorptive surface, leading to impaired absorption of almost all nutrients.[1] Partial or isolated malabsorption results from diseases that interfere with the absorption of specific nutrients.[3]

TYPES OF MALABSORPTION DISORDERS
Luminal and Brush Border Processing Phase

Diseases affecting the luminal phase of the absorption process cause most acquired cases of malabsorption. These include diseases affecting the absorptive surface (**Table 2**), as well as diseases causing digestive enzyme deficiencies.

Short bowel syndrome
Short bowel syndrome is a result of a reduction in intestinal length, usually because of surgery, and is a clinical cause of malabsorption. These intestinal resections lead to decreased absorption of macronutrients and/or water and electrolytes because of insufficient small bowel length. The length and absorptive capacity of the remnant bowel is also contributory.[8] Total small bowel length of less than 200 cm in adults is defined as short bowel syndrome and generally requires nutritional or fluid supplementation.[4,5] Although a universal definition in children has not been developed, short bowel syndrome is assumed when there is a need for intravenous supplementation or when there is a residual small bowel length of less than 25% expected for gestational age.[4,5] The most common causes of short bowel syndrome in adults are Crohn disease, mesenteric ischemia, radiation enteritis, and postoperative complications. In children, intestinal volvulus, malformations, and necrotizing enterocolitis are characteristic.[7,9]

More than 90% of dietary nutrients are absorbed in the jejunum. The ileum compensates but there are permanent changes in enzyme secretion, which may lead to rapid

Table 2
Luminal and brush border processing phase disorders

Entity	Etiologic factors	Specific Diseases
Intestinal resections	Surgical resection <200 cm of small bowel leads to inadequate absorption Absence of Bauhin valve	Short bowel syndrome Bariatric surgery Results in bacterial overgrowth
Intestinal mechanical obstruction	↓ nutrition, ↑ intestinal secretion of fluids and electrolytes in the obstructed segment, ↑ intestinal loss of fluid and electrolytes from nausea or vomiting	Strictures from Crohn Extensive adhesions or peritoneal carcinomas
Intestinal fistulas	Large areas of absorptive mucosal surface are bypassed, resulting in premature loss of nutrients	Crohn Diverticular disease Pancreatic disease Radiation enteritis Colon cancer Ovarian cancer Small bowel cancer
Intestinal dysmotility	Propulsion of contents through intestines in inhibited, without shortening of the length of intestine Acute: impaired motility from intraabdominal inflammation chronic intestinal pseudoobstruction	Ileus diabetes Systemic scleroderma Amyloidosis
Small bowel mucosal disease	Depends in location, severity, and extension of the disease	Crohn Celiac disease Radiation enteritis Autoimmune enteropathy Amyloidosis Giardiasis Tropical sprue Whipple disease

Abbreviations: ↑, increase; ↓, decrease.

gastric emptying.[4,7,9] The ileum secretes protease and carbohydrate enzymes, which are responsible for the breakdown of proteins and carbohydrates. The ileum is also responsible for reabsorbing most daily secretions, such as fatty acids and glycerol. The ileum also is responsible for vitamin B_{12}, bile acids, and magnesium absorption.[1,3,7] Therefore, resections of the ileum result in diarrhea with sodium-chloride and water loss. Fat malabsorption, fat-soluble vitamin deficiency, and B_{12} deficiency may also occur. The smooth muscles of the ileum contract to propel undigested food into the large intestine.

Because the colon's primary functions are fluid and electrolyte absorption and uptake of short-chain fatty acids, small bowel and colon continuity are essential. Resection of the ileocecal valve may allow bacteria from the colon to populate in the small intestine. Because bacteria compete for nutrients with enterocytes, bacterial overgrowth may occur, thereby impeding digestion and absorption.[3,7,10]

There are 3 stages of small bowel syndrome following a surgical procedure: (1) acute stage, (2) adaptation stage, and (3) maintenance stage.[4,10,11]

The acute stage
- Lasts 3 to 4 weeks[4,7]
- Can be life-threatening owing to electrolyte imbalances and dehydration[4,7]
- Often requires parenteral or enteral nutritional support.[4,7]

The adaption stage
- Spontaneous process[4,7]
- Begins 48 hours after resections and takes place over the course of 1 to 2 years[4,7]
- Aimed at increasing surface area and absorption.[4,7]

The maintenance stage
- Absorptive capacity of the intestine is at capacity[4,7]
- Depends on whether the intestinal failure reverses during adaption
  - In reversible failure, patients' nutritional status is maintained through special diets and supplements[4,7]
  - In irreversible failure, patients are destined to lifelong home parenteral nutrition.[4,7]

Small bowel mucosal diseases lead to loss of absorptive mucosal surface, resulting in impaired absorption of almost all nutrients. This impaired absorption can lead to protein-losing enteropathies.

Bariatric surgery induces weight loss in morbidly obese patients by creating malabsorptive defects. The roux-en-Y bypass is the most common method. This results in maldigestion and malabsorption of iron, calcium, magnesium, and folic acid due to a bypassed duodenum. The reduction in the stomach capacity causes reduction in intrinsic factor and a subsequent B_{12} deficiency. Steatorrhea and failed absorption of fat-soluble vitamins D and E also occurs.[3] Patients must be closely monitored for malnutrition, and lifelong vitamin and mineral supplements are recommended.[3,7]

Celiac disease

Celiac disease is a chronic autoimmune disorder. It is caused by both an innate and adaptive immune response to dietary gluten found in wheat, barley, and rye. A genetic component has been associated with the disease. The HLA-DQ2 and/or DQ8 gene loci are found in almost all patients. In celiac disease, gluten proteins are activated by tissue transglutaminase (TTG), which allows it to present to CD4 T cells in the small intestine. Subsequently, cytokines release, resulting in histologic changes in the intestinal mucosa.[7,12,13]

These histologic changes are hallmarks of the disease, including villous atrophy, crypt proliferation, and increased intraepithelial lymphocytes.[7,14] Malabsorption results after villous injury reduces the surface area of the portion of the small bowel needed for absorption, causing impaired production of lactase and other enzymes.[7] Deficiencies in folic acid, iron, and fat-soluble vitamins are common.

Celiac disease is classified as classic, atypical, asymptomatic (silent), and latent.[14,15] Classic disease includes villous atrophy, malabsorption symptoms, and resolution of mucosal lesions after a few weeks to months following the discontinuation of foods with gluten. Patients with classic disease usually present with diarrhea and weight loss.[14,15] Patients with atypical disease have severe mucosal damage but present with minor GI complaints. Abnormal transaminase levels may be the initial finding in some patients.[16] These patients are at risk for significant morbidity due to anemia, osteoporosis, or arthritis. Asymptomatic, or silent, disease is characterized by absence of symptoms. These patients are often diagnosed incidentally. Latent disease occurs either when a patient has fully recovered from celiac after years of consuming a gluten-free diet or when symptoms do not reappear with introduction of a normal diet.[14,15,17]

Crohn disease

Crohn disease is a chronic inflammatory bowel disease that can be remitting and re-lapsing in nature. Inflammation of the small intestines causes damage to the mucosal lining, causing malabsorption. It can affect any part of the GI tract but the small bowel is affected in an estimated 70% of patients with disease and one-third of patients have disease confined to the small bowel.[7,18]

Malabsorption and malnutrition are complications of Crohn disease. Malabsorption in Crohn depends on the portion of bowel affected. In terminal ileum involvement, bile, salt, and B_{12} malabsorption occurs. Vitamin D deficiency also is common in Crohn, resulting in bone disease comorbidities. Malabsorption in Crohn can also result from bowel resections or fistulas. Extensive small bowel mucosal disease leading to loss of absorptive surface could result in malabsorption, steatorrhea, and malnutri-tion.[19] This loss of surface results in impaired absorption of almost all nutrients, mimicking short bowel syndrome.[3,7] Jejunum involvement can lead to protein-energy malnutrition because protein, carbohydrates, and fats are absorbed there.[7]

Surgical resections can lead to short bowel syndrome and chronic intestinal failure. An ileostomy leaves the colon in discontinuity, which can lead to water and electrolyte imbalances. Following ileocecal resection, small intestinal bacterial overgrowth is common.[7,19]

Radiation enteropathy

Radiation enteritis is used to define small intestine injury from radiotherapy.[20] Pelvic and abdominal radiotherapy damage leads to changes in intestinal physiology. Typical changes in bowel tissue include inflammation or cell death of the mucosa, inflamma-tion of the lamina propria, and eosinophilic crypt abscesses.[20] These changes can lead to multiple areas of small bowel dysfunction and/or strictures.[20] Decreased gut motility, nutrient and bile acid malabsorption, and small intestine bacterial overgrowth are clinical features of radiation enteropathy.[20]

Medications

Medications can impair digestion in various ways. Orlistat (Xenical) binds to pancre-atic lipase to impair digestion and absorption for weight loss but can result in fat and fat-soluble vitamin malabsorption.[3,6,7] Nonsteroidal antiinflammatories can cause drug-induced enteropathy.[3] Colchicine (Colcrys) can damage intestinal mu-cosa, causing villous atrophy with general malabsorption or reversible lactase insufficiency.[6]

Human immunodeficiency virus–AIDS

Opportunistic infections seen in AIDS can result in global malabsorption. Human im-munodeficiency virus (HIV) enteropathy can be seen in the absence of these opportu-nistic infections. HIV enteropathy occurs as a result of the virus on the GI tract and the gut-associated lymphoid tissue.[21] Histologic changes may be observed, such as villous atrophy, crypt hyperplasia, and villous blunting to the GI tract. Inflammatory in-filtrates of lymphocytes in the lamina propria may also be observed.[21] Absorption of vitamin B_{12}, fat, and lactose have also been shown to be impaired in patients living with HIV. Although the mechanisms are not entirely known,[6] pathogenic mechanisms of malabsorption in patients with HIV include ileal dysfunction, exudative enteropathy, altered motility, bacterial overgrowth, inflammatory mediators, and secretory enterotoxin.[22]

Absorption into the Intestinal Mucosa

Acquired cases of malabsorption in the mucosal absorptive phase may include a brush border enzyme deficiency, a brush border transport deficiency, or an enterocyte defect.

Lactose intolerance

Lactase is an enzyme present in the brush border membrane of the small intestine. Lactose, hydrolyzed by lactase, is found in mammalian milk. Most humans' lactase activity declines after age 2 to 3 years. Only about 35% can digest lactose beyond the age of 7 to 8 years.[23] Lactose malabsorption refers to low lactase activity without symptoms. Lactose intolerance is defined when the malabsorption causes symptoms.[23]

Inadequate lactase enzyme results in unabsorbed lactose. This unabsorbed lactose travels rapidly into the colon where it is converted to short-chain fatty acids and hydrogen gas by colonic microflora. These byproducts and unfermented lactose cause lactose intolerance symptoms.[23]

Lactase deficiency can be either primary or secondary. Primary lactase deficiency is the most common, consisting of 3 subtypes:

- Primary lactase deficiency
  - Genetic reduction in lactase enzyme activity
  - Most often found in persons of Asian or African descent
- Developmental lactase deficiency
  - Occurs in premature infants
  - Fetal lactase activity develops late in gestation; therefore, babies born between 28 to 32 weeks have a reduction in lactase activity. If otherwise healthy, the colon compensates and symptoms are minimal.
- Congenital lactase deficiency
  - Rare autosomal recessive disorder
  - Absence of lactase activity in the small intestine requiring lactose-free formula.
- Secondary lactase deficiency
  - Occurs due to underlying intestinal disease
  - Examples: small intestinal bacterial overgrowth, intestinal infections, or inflammation as in Crohn, celiac, rotavirus, and radiation enteritis.[3,23] These infections and/or inflammations cause damage to the epithelium, which can result in lactose malabsorption. The lactase enzyme is often the first disaccharide to be affected, presumably because of its distal location on the villus.[3]

Transport into the Circulation

Transport of absorbed nutrients into the general circulation is the final stage of absorption. Lipid transport depends on the lymphatic system. Obstruction in the lymphatic system can impair absorption of lipoproteins and lead to fat malabsorption, steatorrhea, chylous ascites and/or protein-losing enteropathies.[3] Primary intestinal lymphangiectasis, secondary obstructions from lymphoma, and infectious causes such as Whipple disease are all possible causes of lymphatic obstruction.

DIAGNOSIS

Malabsorption disorders are multifactorial, making diagnosis difficult. Symptoms are nonspecific and are frequently mistaken for other conditions, resulting in missed diagnoses. A comprehensive history can often be diagnostic. Several laboratory studies, imaging, and endoscopic evaluations are available to aid in diagnosing malabsorption disorders.

Chronic diarrhea is the most common symptom seen in malabsorption syndromes. Because diarrhea is symptomatic of many illnesses, malabsorption is not always readily considered, which can delay diagnosis and treatment. The history should go beyond the typical problems of timing, frequency, and color to include queries regarding the character of the stool.

Stool Studies

Stools studies are the mainstay of diagnostic evaluation in a patient with persistent diarrhea. The fecal fat test, the van de Kamer method, or the Sudan stain of fecal fat, collected over a 48 to 72 hour period, are used to diagnose fat malabsorption.[2,24] Quantitatively, excretion of more than 7% to 8% of fat diagnoses steatorrhea. Excretion is increased in impaired intraluminal digestion, mucosal disease, and lymphatic obstruction.[24] This test is not frequently ordered because it can be cumbersome. Patients may fail to collect stool accurately or not complete the collection process. For those who have mild steatorrhea, the test may also prove to be ineffective in making a diagnosis.

Stool can also be evaluated for the presence of carbohydrate malabsorption. Although an indirect assessment of carbohydrate malabsorption, the examination of the stool's pH and the osmotic gap may indicate its presence. Examining the feces for pH is not a reliable test because the sensitivity is questionable. However, the specificity of the examination does increase as the pH declines. Due to the potential of ingesting a poorly absorbed substance containing magnesium, sulfate, or phosphate, osmotic gap testing may also lack specificity in regard to carbohydrate malabsorption.[25,26]

Breath Test

Hydrogen breath tests detect the presence of gases produced by colonic bacterial fermentation[2] and are instrumental in detecting carbohydrate malabsorption (lactose, fructose, sucrose, and others), as well as the malabsorption that occurs from small bowel bacterial overgrowth. These tests can also monitor patients during treatment.[26] False negatives and false positives do occur with this form of testing[16,26]:

- False negatives: reduction in breath hydrogen as seen in impaired gastric emptying from diabetic gastroparesis, chronic pulmonary diseases, recent usage of antibiotics, or even absence of hydrogen-producing bacteria[16,26]
- False positives: small bowel bacterial overgrowth.[16]

Laboratory Studies

Although no serologic tests are specific for malabsorption, laboratory studies remain beneficial in the screening and diagnosis of malabsorption. Laboratory findings are often used in conjunction with other diagnostic modalities to provide supportive evidence in arriving at a definitive and firm diagnosis.[26] Laboratory studies should be obtained based on the presentation of symptoms and the suspicion of a particular disease process due to its physiology (**Table 3**).

Imaging Studies

Radiological methods are useful in the diagnosis of malabsorption. The small bowel series was among the initial radiological evaluation methods used in detecting abnormalities of the small intestine.[27] This test has been useful in diagnosing Crohn disease, iron deficiency anemia, unexplained GI bleeding (following upper and lower endoscopy), malabsorption, and diarrhea.[28] However, the small bowel series lacks sensitivity to small mucosal abnormalities of the small intestines.[28] Because of the poor specificity in detecting these abnormalities, computed tomography (CT) enterography has been

Table 3 Laboratory studies in malabsorption syndromes	
Malabsorption Conditions	**Laboratory Studies**
Celiac	Tissue TTG immunoglobulin (Ig)A (screening test) Tissue TTG IgG (screening test) Endomysial IgA (screening test) CBC Iron studies (iron level, TIBC, iron saturation, folate and B12 level) Vitamin C and D levels
Crohn disease	CBC Vitamin B12 Folate Iron studies (iron level, TIBC, iron saturation, folate, and B12 level) CRP
Short bowel syndrome	Proximal ileum evaluation Iron Folate Calcium level Distal ileum evaluation Vitamin B12 level
Radiation enteritis	CBC Iron studies (iron level, TIBC, iron saturation, folate, and B12 level) CMP LFTs PT INR

Abbreviations: CBC, complete blood count; CMP, complete metabolic panel; CRP, C-reactive protein; INR, international normalized ratio; LFTs, liver function test; PT, prothrombin time; TIBC, total iron binding capacity.

used to identify issues concerning the small intestines. According to the American College of Radiology Appropriateness Criteria,[28] CT enterography has become the standard of care in the diagnosis of Crohn disease. It has the benefits of displaying pathologic conditions inside and outside of the bowel with better visualization than the small bowel series. Strictures and obstructions are better visualized and it lacks the concern encountered when using capsule endoscopy. It is also useful in diagnosing celiac disease. CT enterography should be avoided in patients who have an allergy to intravenous contrast material and individuals who have chronic renal insufficiency. Although there are many diagnostic benefits to this test, CT enterography is a costly diagnostic test and may not be used as first-line because of the cost.[28,29]

Endoscopic Evaluation

Endoscopic evaluation has been deemed truly diagnostic for most conditions of the GI tract. Lesions, polyps, strictures, and bleeding can be visualized during the endoscopic evaluation, which aids in diagnosing the underlying cause of malabsorption. Biopsies taken during the endoscopy provide a definitive diagnosis.[26] Although useful, endoscopy with biopsy does have some limitations because complete visualization of the small intestines is not usually possible. Evaluation of the small intestine via endoscopy with biopsy may yield tissue that appears abnormal but histologically lacks specificity, requiring further evaluation.[16] Additional serologic or diagnostic testing, imaging, a trial of medications, or a trial of elimination of particular food from the diet may be necessary. Conversely, the determination of malabsorption can also be associated with a specific lesion found in the small intestines and endoscopy with biopsy alone can be diagnostic.

Wireless capsule endoscopy (WCE) is a procedure in which a pill-structured device equipped with a camera is ingested and later evacuated during a bowel movement. WCE is used to provide direct and complete visualization of the small intestines that is not entirely achievable with conventional endoscopic methods. It is useful in detecting mucosal abnormalities of Crohn and celiac disease. It is often used as part of the trilogy for the diagnoses of anemia: esophagogastroduodenoscopy, colonoscopy, and capsule endoscopy. Although WCE is an excellent diagnostic modality for diagnosing some malabsorption conditions through direct visualization, it lacks the ability to make a tissue diagnosis. Therefore, it is often used in conjunction with endoscopy with biopsy to make a definitive diagnosis. Because of the risk of retention, WCE is used with caution in conditions in which a suspected malignancy or stricturing Crohn disease is suspected.[16,26]

CLINICAL MANAGEMENT AND PROGNOSIS

The specific disease and symptoms guide the treatment of malabsorption syndromes. The comprehensive goals of treatment are

- Treatment of diarrhea and other symptomatology[30]
- Identification and correction of nutritional deficits[30]
- Identification and treatment of underlying disease.[30]

When underlying pathophysiology cannot be completely corrected, management of diarrhea is an important aspect of the treatment plan.[30] Nonspecific antidiarrheal agents, such as loperamide, diphenoxylate with atropine, and deodorized tincture of opium, are used in such cases.[30] Dietary measures, such as a low-fat diet, avoiding caffeine, diluting soft drinks and fruit juices with water by a 1-to-1 ratio, and oral rehydration for severe diarrhea are also helpful.[30] In patients with fat malabsorption, exogenous conjugated bile acid therapy can decrease steatorrhea. Nutrient supplementation depends on the type of malabsorption.

Short Bowel Syndrome

Prompt reversal of dehydration and nutritional deficiency should be initiated in short bowel syndrome. Intravenous fluids are given to correct problems associated with dehydration. Replacement of vitamin and minerals typically resolve nutritional deficiencies. Proton pump inhibitors help with acid secretory functions because issues regarding acid secretion are contributory factors in malabsorption associated with short bowel syndrome. Medications such as loperamide slow down motility, therefore increasing contact time of nutrients in the small intestine, improving absorption, and treating diarrhea.[31–33] In an effort to reduce the amount of atrophy and maximize mucosal hyperplasia, enteral feedings are started early, whereas total parental nutrition (TPN) is a last resort in treatment.[16] Concomitant treatment with teduglutide, a long-acting homolog of the hormone GLP-2, has been associated with improved intestinal absorption, therefore reducing the amount of TPN required.[30] Lifelong side effects of short bowel syndrome often derive from the underlying disease, altered bowel anatomy and physiology, or the treatment. However, with short bowel syndrome, individuals can live a healthy life with symptom control and nutrient supplementation. Over time, the body may adapt to having a smaller than usual length of intestines thereby causing symptoms to lessen and potential nutritional deficiencies to be averted.[34,35] In the case of chronic irreversible short bowel syndrome, small intestinal transplantation can be performed.[34,35]

Celiac Disease

The approach to treating celiac disease is twofold. Individuals with celiac disease have a gluten sensitivity that makes ingestion of gluten-containing foods hazardous. Elimination of these products from the diet is necessary to resolve symptoms and avoid disease progression. Anemia and osteopenia are common clinical manifestations of celiac disease that occur due to malabsorption of iron, folate, and vitamins C and D.[36] Iron supplementation should be started if iron deficiency anemia is present. Refractory anemia that remains after 1 to 2 years of a gluten-free diet requires swift intravenous iron therapy replacement. If osteopenia is suspected, bone density testing should be done to assess the full extent of the condition. Calcium and vitamin D supplementation should also be started.[37] The prognosis of celiac disease is usually uneventful. Individuals who are symptomatic with years of gluten exposure are more prone to developing lymphoma. There is also a small probability that small GI and pharyngeal carcinomas can develop in those with celiac disease. Therefore, strict elimination of gluten-containing foods and beverages is beneficial in reducing the risk of these conditions.[16]

Crohn Disease

The goal of treatment in Crohn disease is to achieve remission. This is accomplished with mucosal healing therapies, as well as replacing nutrients lost due to the malabsorption that occurs with the disease process.[38] Medications that heal the mucosal lining in Crohn disease include 5-aminosalicylates, budesonide, thiopurines, and anti-tumor necrosis factor biologic agents.[22] Similar to the use of corticosteroids in the management of an acute flare, budesonide can be used in the same manner (**Table 4**).[38,39] Surgery is reserved for complicated, fistulizing, and stricturing disease states. Surgery, however, is not curative because reoccurrences are common. Crohn disease prognosis is associated with an increased risk of developing colon cancer. Therefore, surveillance with colonoscopies are recommended every 1 to 2 years after having the disease for more than 8 years.[40]

Radiation Enteritis

The treatment of radiation enteritis encompasses treatment of bacterial overgrowth with antibiotics if present. Bile salts-binding medications are used to control bile salt–induced diarrhea. TPN and dietary supplements can be used as supportive measures.[16]

The prognosis in patients who have radiation enteritis is capricious because the condition is considered progressive. Reoccurrence of cancer decreases survival of those with radiation enteritis. Patients often have GI symptoms for the rest of their lives.[41] Surgery is indicated in individuals who, despite treatment, continue to have severe intestinal or colonic strictures, fistulas, and symptoms (see **Table 4**). Surgery is associated with a high rate of death because the circulation needed for healing is impaired due to the affected intestine.[16]

Lactose Intolerance

Lactose intolerance does not always require complete elimination of dietary lactose. Restriction to 2 cups of milk or milk products daily taken with 2 meals may be sufficient to treat symptoms. Lactose-reduced products or lactase supplements are also

Table 4
Treatment and prognosis of malabsorption conditions

Malabsorption Condition	Treatment	Prognosis

Celiac disease	Discontinuation of gluten
	  Wheat
	  Barley
	  Rye
	  Triticale
	Anemia
	  Oral or intravenous iron
	  Folate
	Osteopenia
	  Vitamin C and D
	    supplementation
		Excellent in most cases
		↑ incidence of intestinal lymphoma in symptomatic patients with years of gluten exposure
		↑ incidence of small intestinal, esophageal, and pharyngeal carcinomas with years of gluten exposure and symptomatic patients

Crohn Disease	Flare rescue
	  Corticosteroids
	  Budesonide
	Remission (induction or maintenance)
	  5-aminosalicylate
	  Thiopurines
	  Antitumor necrosis factor
	Induction of remission
	  Budesonide
		Overall good prognosis
		Indolent course
		Fistulizing or stricturing Crohn requiring resection
		Relapses and remission
		Colorectal cancer

Short Bowel Syndrome	Immediate intravenous fluid resuscitation Nutrient supplementation Proton pump inhibitors Loperamide ↓ motility or ↑ absorption TPN	Life-long side effects ↓ in symptoms as body adapts and nutritional deficiencies averted
Radiation Enteropathy	Antibiotic for bacterial overgrowth (if applicable) Bile salts medication for diarrhea TPN	Surgery for stricture or fistulas Death
Lactose Intolerance	Elimination of lactose-containing products	Excellent with restrictions of lactose in diet
HIV Enteropathy	Highly active antiretroviral therapy (HAART) Nutritional supplementation Electrolytes Symptom control	HAART is usually effective

beneficial. Calcium replacement may be necessary in patients with inadequate intake. Vitamin D levels should be monitored.[23,42]

Human Immunodeficiency Virus–AIDS Enteropathy

Highly active antiretroviral therapy (HAART), damaging effects of HIV on the GI system, HIV-causing malignancies, and pancreatitis are all causes of diarrhea seen in the HIV-infected patient.[21] Before initiating treatment of diarrhea, an infectious process and other causes of diarrhea must be ruled out to arrive at the diagnosis of HIV-AIDS enteropathy. Diagnosing and treating this condition is complex and may require an interprofessional team.[43] Treatment is mostly supportive and involves

- Starting and managing HAART
- Providing nutritional supplementation
- Replacing electrolytes
- Initiating symptom-controlling medications.[42]

Highly active antiretroviral medications usually improve the symptoms of HIV enteropathy. There are cases in which it is not always effective.[43]

SUMMARY

Symptoms that are associated with common illnesses often mimic those of malabsorption. These symptoms are frequently associated with illnesses of viral origin, medication side effects, or even parasitic infections, with little consideration given to diseases of the small intestines. Therefore, diagnosis and treatment of malabsorption can be delayed or missed. Subsequently, treatment is focused primarily on symptom control and not disease management. Malabsorption syndromes may arise from multiple modalities, with small intestine disorders being the leading cause. Although gastroenterologists are keenly involved in the diagnosis and treatment of malabsorption, primary care providers are also instrumental in early detection, testing, and treatment of malabsorption-causing disorders. It is essential for primary care providers to be able to readily identify symptoms associated with malabsorption so that diagnosis and treatment can occur early, thus averting suffering and complications.

REFERENCES

1. Keller J, Layer P. The pathophysiology of malabsorption. Visc Med 2014;30(3): 150–4.
2. Nikaki K, Gupte GL. Assessment of intestinal malabsorption. Best Pract Res Clin Gastroenterol 2016;30(2):225–35.
3. van der Heide F. Acquired causes of intestinal malabsorption. Best Pract Res Clin Gastroenterol 2016;30(2):213–24.
4. Pironi L. Definitions of intestinal failure and the short bowel syndrome. Best Pract Res Clin Gastroenterol 2016;30(2):173–85.
5. Pironi L, Arends J, Bozzetti F, et al. ESPEN guidelines on chronic intestinal failure in adults. Clin Nutr 2016;35(2):247–307.
6. Montalto M, Santoro L, D'Onofrio F, et al. Classification of malabsorption syndromes. Dig Dis 2008;26(2):104–11.
7. Nolan JD, Johnston IM, Walters JRF. Physiology of malabsorption. Surgery 2015; 33(5):193–9.
8. Tappenden KA. Pathophysiology of short bowel syndrome considerations of resected and residual anatomy. JPEN J Parenter Enteral Nutr 2014;38: 14S–22S.
9. Uchino M, Ikeuchi H, Bando T, et al. Risk factors for short bowel syndrome in patients with Crohn's disease. Surg Today 2012;42(5):447–52.
10. Cagir B, Sawyer M. Short-bowel syndrome. 2017. Available at: https://emedicine.medscape.com/article/193391-overview. Accessed March 18, 2018.
11. Sundaram A, Koutkia P, Apovian CM. Nutritional management of short bowel syndrome in adults. J Clin Gastroenterol 2002;34(3):207–20.
12. Goebel SU. Celiac disease (Sprue). 2017. Available at: https://emedicine.medscape.com/article/171805-overview. Accessed March 20, 2018.
13. Green PHR, Lebwohl B, Greywoode R. Celiac disease. J Allergy Clin Immunol 2015;135(5):1099–106.

14. Hill I. Epidemiology, pathogenesis, and clinical manifestations of celiac disease in children. 2018. Available at: https://www.uptodate.com/contents/epidemiology-pathogenesis-and-clinical-manifestations-of-celiac-disease-in-children. Accessed March 20, 2018.
15. Tonutti E, Bizzaro N. Diagnosis and classification of celiac disease and gluten sensitivity. Autoimmun Rev 2014;13(4):472–6.
16. Trier JS. Intestinal malabsorption. In: Greenberger NJ, Blumberg RS, Burakoff R, editors. CURRENT diagnosis & treatment: gastroenterology, hepatology, & endoscopy, 3e. New York: McGraw-Hill; 2016. Available at: http://accessmedicine.mhmedical.com.ezproxy.uthsc.edu/content.aspx?bookid=1621&sectionid=105183794. Accessed March 23, 2018.
17. Dewar DH, Ciclitira PJ. Clinical features and diagnosis of celiac disease. Gastroenterology 2005;128(4):S19–24.
18. Leighton JA, Pasha SF. Inflammatory diseases of the small bowel. Gastrointest Endosc Clin N Am 2017;27(1):63–77.
19. Gajendran M, Loganathan P, Catinella AP, et al. A comprehensive review and update on Crohn's disease. Dis Mon 2018;64(2):20–57.
20. Stacey R, Green JT. Radiation-induced small bowel disease: latest developments and clinical guidance. Ther Adv Chronic Dis 2014;5(1):15–29.
21. Macarthur RD, Dupont HL. Etiology and pharmacologic management of noninfectious diarrhea in HIV-infected individuals in the highly active antiretroviral therapy era. Clin Infect Dis 2012;55(6):860–7.
22. Lu SS. Pathophysiology of HIV-associated diarrhea. Gastroenterol Clin North Am 1997;26(2):175–89.
23. Hurduc V, Bordei L, Plesca V, et al. OC-30 Lactose intolerance: new aspects of an old problem. Arch Dis Child 2017;102(Suppl 2):A11–2.
24. Hawkey C. Textbook of clinical gastroenterology and hepatology [e-book]. Chichester (England): Wiley-Blackwell; 2012. Available from: eBook Collection (EBSCOhost). Accessed March 24, 2018.
25. Mason JB, Milovic V. Clinical features and diagnosis of malabsorption. 2017, Available at: https://www.uptodate.com/contents/clinical-features-and-diagnosis-of-malabsorption#H3. Accessed March 15, 2018.
26. Pollack MS. ACR practice parameter for the performance of a barium small bowel examination in adults. 2013;1–7.
27. Baker ME. ACR practice parameter for the performance of computer tomography (CT) enterography. 2015;1–13.
28. Panes J, Bouhnik Y, Reinisch W, et al. Imaging techniques for assessment of inflammatory bowel disease: joint ECCO and ESGAR evidence-based consensus guidelines. J Crohns Colitis 2013;7(7):556–85.
29. Mason JB, Milovic V. Overview of the treatment of malabsorption. 2016; Available at: https://www.uptodate.com/contents/overview-of-the-treatment-of-malabsorption?search=lactose%20intolerance&source=search_result&selectedTitle=4~150&usage_type=default&display_rank=4#H6. Accessed March 21, 2018.
30. DiBaise JK. Pathophysiology of short bowel syndrome. UpToDate. Available at: https://www.uptodate.com/contents/pathophysiology-of-short-bowel-syndrome#! Accessed March 23, 2018.
31. DiBaise JK. Management of the short bowel syndrome in adults. Waltham (MA): UpToDate; 2017. Available at: https://www.uptodate.com/contents/management-of-the-short-bowel-syndrome-in-adults. Accessed March 24, 2018.
32. Schulzke J-D, Tröger H, Amasheh M. Disorders of intestinal secretion and absorption. Best Pract Res Clin Gastroenterol 2009;23(3):395–406.

33. Kelly DG, Tappenden KA, Winkler MF. Short bowel syndrome. JPEN J Parenter Enteral Nutr 2013;38(4):427–37.
34. Tappenden KA. Intestinal adaptation following resection. JPEN J Parenter Enteral Nutr 2014;38(1 suppl):23S–31S.
35. Schuppan D. Pathogenesis, epidemiology, and clinical manifestations of celiac disease in adults. Waltham (MA): UpToDate; 2016. Available at: https://www.uptodate.com/contents/pathogenesis-epidemiology-and-clinical-manifestations-of-celiac-disease-in-adults. Accessed March 24, 2018.
36. Stein J, Connor S, Virgin G, et al. Anemia and iron deficiency in gastrointestinal and liver conditions. World J Gastroenterol 2016;22(35):1–29.
37. Regueiro M, Rutgeerts P, Robosn KM. Overview of the medical management of mild (low risk) Crohn disease in adults. UpToDate; 2018. Available at: https://www.uptodate.com/contents/overview-of-the-medical-management-of-mild-low-risk-crohn-disease-in-adults. Accessed March 24, 2018.
38. Kuenzig ME, Rezaie A, Otley AR, et al. Budesonide for maintenance of remission in Crohn's disease (Review). Cochrane Libr 2014;(8):1–200.
39. Levine JS, Burakoff R. Inflammatory bowel disease: medical considerations. In: Greenberger NJ, Blumberg RS, Burakoff R, editors. CURRENT diagnosis & treatment: gastroenterology, hepatology, & endoscopy, 3e. New York: McGrawHill; Available at: http://accessmedicine.mhmedical.com.ezproxy.uthsc.edu/content.aspx?bookid=1621&sectionid=105181325. Accessed March 23, 2018.
40. Roberts I. Diagnosis and management of chronic radiation enteritis. UpToDate; 2016. Available at: https://www.uptodate.com/contents/diagnosis-and-management-of-chronic-radiation-enteritis#!. Accessed March 24, 2018.
41. Hammer HF, Hogenauer C. Lactose intolerance: Clinical manifestations, diagnosis, and management. 2018. Available at: https://www.uptodate.com/contents/lactose-intolerance-clinical-manifestations-diagnosis-and-management?search=lactose%20intolerance&source=search_result&selectedTitle=1~150&usage_type=default&display_rank=1#H17. Accessed March 20, 2018.
42. Cello JP, Day LW. Idiopathic AIDS enteropathy and treatment of gastrointestinal opportunistic pathogens. Gastroenterology 2009;136(6):1952–65.
43. Hall VP. Common gastrointestinal complications associated with human immunodeficiency virus/AIDS. Crit Care Nurs Clin North Am 2018;30(1):101–7.

An Overview of Munchausen Syndrome and Munchausen Syndrome by Proxy

Brittany Abeln, BSN, RN*, Rene Love, PhD, DNP, PMHNP-BC

KEYWORDS

- Munchausen syndrome • Munchausen syndrome by proxy • Factitious disorder
- Diagnosis • Treatment

KEY POINTS

- Munchausen syndrome is complex in its diagnosis owing to the nature of its presentation.
- However, an unusual presentation of illness and lack of response to treatment can function as clinical red flags.
- Munchausen syndrome by proxy is the imposed presentation of false illness on another and, although rare, when seen, commonly occurs as childhood abuse with the caregiver functioning as abuser.
- The use of an interdisciplinary team aids in the diagnosis of both Munchausen syndrome and Munchausen syndrome by proxy.
- Early diagnosis is key to aid in the initiation of treatment and intervention.

Munchausen syndrome and Munchausen syndrome by proxy may be notorious in nature, but they are rare and difficult to diagnosis. Munchausen syndrome involves the fabrication of an injury or illness to oneself. Even though it is difficult to identify, Munchausen syndrome presents in approximately 1.3% of all hospitalized patients.[1,2] Alternatively, Munchausen syndrome by proxy involves the fabrication of injury or illness inflicted by 1 person on another (usually parent to child) and accounts for roughly 0.04% of child abuse cases.[1,3] Although uncommon, both conditions are precursors to significant morbidity and mortality. Whether the harm is directed to the self or to another, these syndromes are forms of abuse with long-term psychiatric consequences.

In all its various and accepted spellings—Münchhausen, Münchausen, Munchhausen and Munchausen—this syndrome has been associated with various portrayals in film and other media.[4] The HBO documentary, *Mommy Dead and Dearest* explores the

There are no commercial or financial relationships to disclose.
University of Arizona, College of Nursing, 1305 N. Martin Avenue, Tucson, AZ 85721, USA
* Corresponding author.
E-mail address: babeln@email.arizona.edu

case of Deedee Blanchard and Gypsey Rose, in which Blanchard engages in Munchausen syndrome by proxy with her daughter Gypsey. Even though Gypsey presented with cancer symptoms among other ailments up into her late teens, she was physically healthy. Gypsey ultimately killed her mother after years of abuse were inflicted upon her.

The term Munchausen syndrome was first coined by Dr Richard Alan John Asher in 1951 and named after Hieronymous Carl Fredrich Freiherr von Munchhausen, who also known as Baron von Munchhausen.[4] Baron von Munchhausen was an 18th-century storyteller known for his wild retellings of his exaggerated exploits.[4] Dr Asher noted that those with Munchausen syndrome lied about or embellished their symptoms very similar to the tales by Baron von Munchhausen, thus naming the diagnosis, Munchausen syndrome.[4] In 1977, Sir Samuel Roy Meadow expanded on Dr Asher's work when he recognized that individuals (often caregivers) could falsify injury or illness in others and thus coined the term Munchausen syndrome by proxy.[4]

Although Munchausen syndrome and Munchausen syndrome by proxy are the most commonly used terminologies, other names have been associated with the disorders. Munchausen is recognized as factitious disorder, factitious disorder imposed on self, or fabricated illness. Munchausen syndrome by proxy also is known as induced illness, factitious disorder imposed on others, or caregiver-fabricated illness. The medical terminology used in the *Diagnostic Statistical Manual of Mental Health Disorders, fifth edition* (DSM-5) is factitious disorder imposed on self (Munchausen syndrome) and factitious disorder imposed on another (Munchausen syndrome by proxy).[1]

MUNCHAUSEN SYNDROME
Diagnostic Criteria

As mentioned, Munchausen syndrome according to the DSM-5 is known as factitious disorder imposed on self.[1] (See the DSM-5 criteria for factitious disorder imposed on self). It is important to note, when diagnosing a patient, whether this is a single episode of Munchausen syndrome or reoccurring instances.[1] This disorder usually presents at the onset of adulthood and it is often identified through atypical presentations that are not supported through clinical examination including but not limited to laboratory tests, scans, and physical examination. Additional considerations for the diagnosis of Munchausen syndrome include a history of multiple past health care services with unsuccessful treatment and an individual who has an unusual foundation of medical knowledge.[1,5]

Common Features of the Patient

When diagnosing Munchausen syndrome, the health care provider must consider common features in patient presentations. **Box 1** lists common characteristics of the individual with Munchausen syndrome. The common characteristics are not inclusive of all individual presentations with Munchausen syndrome; however, they are characteristic of common features representing identified patients. There may be a myriad of other possible characteristics outside of the common features listed in the table, so it is important to address concerns as they arise based on the history and physical examination.

How to Diagnose

There are many clinical red flags or suspicious behaviors that may alert medical professionals to suspect a diagnosis of Munchausen syndrome. **Box 2** identifies such

---

Box 1
Common characteristics of the individual with Munchausen syndrome

Female

Health care/laboratory profession

Middle aged (35–50 years old)

Unmarried

Diagnosis of depression

Data from Sadock BJ, Sadock VA, Ruiz P, editors. Kaplan & Sadock's synopsis of psychiatry behavioral science/clinical psychiatry. Lippincott Williams & Wilkins; 2015; and Yates GP, Feldman MD. Factitious disorder: a systematic review of 455 cases in the professional literature. Gen Hosp Psychiatry 2016;41:20–8.

---

common suspicious behavior. One reason a diagnosis can be difficult to formulate is that the individual may be complaining of symptoms of actual concern. Therefore, it is important to obtain a detailed history and physical examination to treat the current symptom presentation. In addition to the treatment of symptoms, addressing the potential diagnosis of Munchausen syndrome when these red flags present themselves is equally important.

Organ Failure

There may be presentations of Munchausen syndrome in which the individual is causing actual harm to themselves.[3] In that case, there may be genuine symptomatology that aligns with the clinical presentation. On occasion, Munchausen syndrome may be suspected if the individual is healthy and, therefore, has no basis for the underlying presenting symptoms based on the history and complete physical examination. The presenting symptoms are seen as questionable and not logical to the provider or treatment team, thus causing concern. In extreme cases, organ failure may result as the symptoms progress.[3]

Treatment Recommendations

When Munchausen syndrome is suspected, the health care provider should avoid accusatory questions and refer the patient for a psychiatric evaluation.[3] However,

---

Box 2
Common red flags of Munchausen syndrome

Unusual presentation of symptoms

Symptoms unresponsive to treatment

Multiple reported drug allergies

Few visitors in an inpatient setting

New symptoms present when previous symptoms subside

Extensive medical history not supported by diagnosis or medical procedures

Data from Sadock BJ, Sadock VA, Ruiz P, editors. Kaplan & Sadock's synopsis of psychiatry behavioral science/clinical psychiatry. Lippincott Williams & Wilkins; 2015; and Yates GP, Feldman MD. Factitious disorder: a systematic review of 455 cases in the professional literature. Gen Hosp Psychiatry 2016;41:20–8.

---

presenting the idea of a psychiatric evaluation is often upsetting; therefore, the patient should be involved in the process. The rationale for the psychiatric consult should be explained to the patient so the individual does not feel like they are being ignored by the treatment team and passed along to psychiatry.

It is important to understand that an individual with Munchausen syndrome may not understand the rationale behind their diagnosis and may not believe they suffer from Munchausen syndrome. When informing the patient that a psychiatric provider will be consulted for an evaluation, the provider should remain positive and caring. The treatment team's overall goal of the promotion of health and well-being in the patient should be communicated to the patient. It is best to avoid telling the patient that the team suspects they have Munchausen syndrome until a diagnosis is confirmed. Before confirmation of the diagnosis, the provider should not abruptly discharge a patient once Munchausen syndrome is suspected. Discharging the patient from the hospital will not ultimately benefit the patient because the behavior patterns may continue.[3] This tactic also applies to the primary care setting—when a diagnosis of Munchausen syndrome is suspected, the provider should be sure not to dismiss the patient, but rather be sure to address the concern.

Once a diagnosis is confirmed, it is important to address the underlying emotional needs of the patient to ascertain the motivation for Munchausen syndrome; the patient may not fully comprehend the new diagnosis.[3] Although no specific therapy has been found to be effective in treating Munchausen syndrome, a focus on management rather than a cure is important.[3] The individual will need to work on developing and refining coping skills to assist in the management of the disorder. The priority in the management of the disease focuses on allowing the individual to recognize when they feel compelled to engage in Munchausen syndrome symptomatology and prevent it from recurring.

Case Study 1

The following fictional case study illuminates how an individual with Munchausen syndrome may present. There are many clinical red flags for a Munchausen syndrome diagnosis within the case study.

Patient A is a 33-year-old woman who presents to the emergency department (ED) complaining of stomach pain. She states that she has been having diffuse stomach pain for the past day and a half with nausea, vomiting, and diarrhea. Patient A lists several allergies—phenergan, morphine, vancomycin, hydrocodone, and diphenhydramine (Benadryl). She arrived at the ED alone with no family or friends accompanying her. Upon taking a medical history from patient A, the staff discover that she has a significant, lengthy health history; she has made 7 visits to the ED over the past 6 months. She reports a history of fibromyalgia, gastroesophageal reflux disease, and asthma. She was diagnosed with asthma as a child and had many trips to the hospital related to exacerbations of the illness.

Patient A is pleasant with hospital staff and in fact seems to enjoy the attention she receives from them. She complains of nausea and wretches often until given medication, which improves the symptoms. Patient A describes her stomach pain as unbearable until given pain medication. An ultrasound examination is performed on her abdomen to assist in determining the cause for her symptoms; the results are within normal limits.

Patient A is told that her ultrasound examination is normal and the suspected diagnosis is food poisoning given the duration of her symptoms. The staff tell patient A they will begin the process of discharging her home after she finishes receiving her intravenous fluids to rehydrate her. Hearing this, she becomes visibly agitated and upset saying that staff are not listening to her and do not want to help her. One provider in the ED sits down with her to discuss what has been going on in patient A's personal life and how her mental state has been. The provider makes a referral to the psychiatric team to come meet and talk with patient A because Munchausen syndrome is suspected.

MUNCHAUSEN SYNDROME BY PROXY
Diagnostic Criteria

Munchausen syndrome by proxy according to the DSM-5 is also known as factitious disorder imposed on another.[1] (See DSM-5 diagnostic criteria for factitious disorder imposed on another).

As with Munchausen syndrome, the diagnosis can be for either a single episode or recurrent episodes of Munchausen syndrome by proxy and might be precipitated by hospitalization of the child.[1] This syndrome occurs in approximately 0.05 to 2.0 per 100,000 children younger than 16 years old.[6] The median age of the child is between 14 months and 2.7 years old when the caregiver is diagnosed.[6] It is very uncommon to see a victim older than 6 years of age.[7]

Common Features of the Perpetrator

Understanding the common characteristics present in both the perpetrating and non-perpetrating parent can help in the identification of Munchausen by proxy. Although either caregiver can be the perpetrator, it is often, the child's mother that is involved in this syndrome.[8] **Box 3** lists the common characteristics of perpetrators of Munchausen syndrome by proxy.

Given that the parent most commonly found to be the perpetrator is the child's mother, it is important to consider if there is a presence of a nonperpetrating caregiver or spouse. The nonperpetrating caregivers/spouses are often distant to or uninvolved with the actions against the child, with marital problems existing within the family.[7,11,12] The nonperpetrating individuals rarely visit the hospital and commonly are busy with work.[7] They also may be aggressive with hospital personnel in contrast with the perpetrator, who tends to be agreeable with staff.[7]

As discussed, Munchausen syndrome by proxy most commonly presents with the victim's mother as the perpetrator. However, there is evidence in older literature that discusses the rare incidence of the father as the perpetrator.[13,14] In a study that

---

Box 3
Common characteristics of perpetrators of Munchausen syndrome by proxy

Female (often the victim's mother)

Childhood abuse

History of Munchausen syndrome

Personality sisorder

Lack of support/disengagement from other parent

Often well-educated

Rarely leave the bedside of child/victim

Develops close relationship with hospital staff

Data from Refs.[7–10]

examined 15 families in which Munchausen syndrome by proxy occurred with the father as the perpetrator, there were some commonalities identified.[13] The father perpetrators commonly presented with histories of their own Munchausen syndrome.[13] The perpetrating fathers were often seen as overbearing and demanding by hospital staff, as well.[13] Interestingly enough, in 4 of the 15 cases examined, unusual fires occurred in the homes.[13] Another 4 of the 15 cases had dogs or cats die in unusual circustances.[13] It is important to note that the fires and unusual deaths may not be indicative of the perpetrating fathers, but rather are notable commonalities.

In a systematic review of 796 cases of Munchausen System by proxy, 96.7% of perpetrators were found to be females and 3.3% were found to be male.[14] Of the perpetrators examined, 91.2% were the victim's mother, 2.9% were the father, and 5.8% had some other relationship with the victim.[14] This systematic review demonstrates the rarity of fathers and males as perpetrators.

Munchausen syndrome by proxy commonly occurs with the parent as perpetrator and their child as victim.[11] However, it is important to clarify that Munchausen syndrome by proxy can also occur with an adult as the victim, seen in circumstances of adult caregiving, for instance, an adult child taking care of their elderly parent.[15,16] Therefore, it is important to be aware of signs and symptoms of Munchausen syndrome by proxy in any patient, at any age, who is dependent on another for care.

Clinical Red Flags or Characteristics

There are common identifying signs and symptoms of Munchausen syndrome by proxy. **Box 4** lists potential symptoms as seen in each body system. Organ failure with concomitant mortality may occur depending on the severity of symptoms and timeliness of diagnosis.[3]

Complicating the diagnosis of Munchausen syndrome by proxy is the victim's presentation with symptoms of real conditions or illnesses, with a diagnosis impacts 1 or more systems. However, the objective data do not substantiate the diagnosis. Therefore, the treatment team needs to be aware of common red flags that exist for Munchausen syndrome by proxy, as identified in **Box 5**.

The common red flags as listed in **Box 5** can assist in detecting Munchausen syndrome by proxy given the nature of presentation of symptoms that is unsubstantiated by the physical examination and history. Although these are common concerns in Munchausen syndrome by proxy, it is important to remember that the victims or caregivers may present with their own set of unique characteristics. Anytime there is a suspicion of the diagnosis based on these and/or other red flags, it should prompt further investigation to rule out a diagnosis of Munchausen syndrome by proxy.

Box 4
Possible symptoms by system of Munchausen syndrome by proxy

Musculoskeletal	Limping, broken bones, muscle weakness
Nervous	Seizures, headaches
Respiratory	Sleep apnea, respiratory distress, asthma, hypoxia
Endocrine	Diabetes
Digestive	Nausea/vomiting, abdominal pain, diarrhea, weight loss, disorders requiring parenteral nutrition
Urinary	Urinary tract infections
Integumentary	Rash, ecchymosis, wounds

Data from Flaherty EG, MacMillan HL, Committee on Child Abuse and Neglect. Caregiver-fabricated illness in a child: a manifestation of child maltreatment. Pediatrics 2013;132(3):590–7.

Box 5
Common red flags of Munchausen syndrome by proxy
Caregiver is not satisfied with the treatment
Symptoms do not correlate with medical findings
Victim does not respond to treatment
Inconsistent patient histories
Symptoms begin in presence of caregiver
Sibling of victim also has unusual symptoms
Caregiver publicly asks for sympathy or donations
Caregiver does not express relief when victim's symptoms or condition improves
Symptomatology seems atypical
Data from Flaherty EG, MacMillan HL, Committee on Child Abuse and Neglect. Caregiver-fabricated illness in a child: a manifestation of child maltreatment. Pediatrics 2013;132(3):590–7; and Yates G, Bass B. The perpetrators of medical child abuse (Munchausen syndrome by proxy)–a systematic review of 796 cases. Child Abuse Negl 2017;72:45–53.

How to Diagnose

To diagnosis Munchausen syndrome by proxy, the treatment team must connect the perplexing way in which the victim presents in conjunction with the behavior of the perpetrator. This process will of course begin as a suspicion, but to confirm the diagnosis there needs to be viable evidence. The use of audio and video surveillance is common to gather definitive data when Munchausen syndrome by proxy is suspected.[17] It is crucial that a multidisciplinary approach involving doctors, nursing staff, social work, legal staff, and hospital security be coordinated when attempting to confirm a diagnosis of Munchausen syndrome by proxy.[17] It is possible that staff or providers can be witness to behavior that incriminates the perpetrator and indicates Munchausen syndrome by proxy. In an attempt to make a definitive diagnosis, it is important to know that it is rare that the victim will indicate that the perpetrator is the cause of the medical symptoms. Once all of the evidence has been obtained, the team can formulate a credible diagnosis that the perpetrator has been causing the symptoms experienced by the victim, thus confirming Munchausen syndrome by proxy.

Organ Failure

The diagnosis of Munchausen syndrome by proxy is complicated by the fact that the victim can present with a complex system issue leading to organ failure. If early diagnosis does not occur, the victim is at risk for their health continuing to deteriorate. Consequently, a missed diagnosis may ultimately lead to organ failure and even death.

Treatment Recommendations

Many cases of Munchausen syndrome by proxy go undiagnosed until the case ends with a fatality. The exact number of fatalities that occur owing to Munchausen syndrome by proxy is difficult to determine because of underreporting and individuals being undiagnosed.[18] Although it is essential that a diagnosis be established as soon as possible to prevent any further unnecessary harm, the average time frame from the onset of symptoms to a reported diagnosis is between 14.9 and 21.8 months.[19] Delay in diagnosis is likely due to the use of multiple tests and procedures, doctor shopping, and the medical professionals' desire to find a medical cause.[17] The perpetrator may decide to move from one provider to the next if the provider does not escalate treatment to the victim. The move to a new provider is the desire to find a provider who will provide extensive, dedicated care as sought after by the perpetrator, despite the lack of objective clinical data.[17]

If the victim is a child, child protective services should be notified; however, if the victim is an adult, then adult protective services is notified after a definitive diagnosis is confirmed. The severity of the injuries may also result in the perpetrator being charged with a crime and possibly serving jail time. Given that Munchausen syndrome by proxy presents as child abuse or elder abuse, separation from the perpetrator and victim must occur for the safety of the victim. This separation is to prevent future harm to the victim. Once separated, the victim can begin to heal while the perpetrator seeks treatment to determine the underlying rationale for their behavior. The child victim will have a guardian enlisted for future medical decisions during the time of separation.[3]

It is important for both the victim and the perpetrator to seek the physical and mental health treatment necessary for healing.[3] Family therapy might also be an option for child victims and parent perpetrators, depending on the severity of the injury.[3] The process of recovery requires an interprofessional team of providers that communicate on a regular basis to promote family wellness.

Reunification between the perpetrator and the victim can occur, but it requires the perpetrator to acknowledge the induced illness and seek treatment.[8] If reunification were to occur, family therapy for all members of the family (perpetrator, nonperpetrator, victim, and siblings) would be crucial to ensure positive relationships moving forward. Family therapy would also ensure that the victim properly heals from the mental consequences, in addition to the physical consequences. Additionally, it would address the need for the perpetrator to use proper coping skills when they have the urge to induce physical symptoms in the victim.

The need for early diagnosis is evident when one examines the possible disturbing outcome of Munchausen syndrome by proxy. In the systematic review of 796 cases, 6.5% of perpetrators gained financially from the abuse of their victim and 35.6% of the victims were subjected to extensive health care as a result of the abuse.[14] Approximately 7.4% of the perpetrators lead to the death of their victim as a result of their abuse, with school attendance being disrupted in 12.3% of the cases reviewed.[14] These are just a few of the possible outcomes of Munchausen syndrome by proxy with the data supporting early detection and diagnosis to lessen the impact on the victim.

Case Study 2

The following fictional case study demonstrates how an individual with Munchausen syndrome by proxy may present. In the example of this case study, a mother with Munchausen syndrome by proxy and her young son presents as the victim.

Ms. R accompanies her son, patient D, age 5 during his hospitalization for seizures. During the week patient D has been hospitalized, he has had 3 seizures. The pediatric team is trying to determine the cause of his seizures. Ms. R never leaves her son's side and is very involved in his care. She always asks for updates from the treatment team and at times is overbearing. Ms. R is a single mom and patient D's father is not involved. Patient D is a very sweet boy and has a great temperament.

The treatment team is having a difficult time determining the cause of patient D's seizures. The team was in the process of discharging patient D to home with seizure medication, when patient D had a fourth seizure. Ms. R insisted that patient D could not leave the hospital until the team figured out what was causing the seizures. The next morning patient D's nurse was entering his room and saw Ms. R touching patient D's IV line. When the nurse asked what Ms. R was doing, Ms. R moved something under the blanket, threw her hands up, and said she was just looking at it.

The nurse later returns to the room and sits to talk with Ms. R about how Ms. R has been handling patient D's illness. Ms. R becomes very defensive and says that she does not want to talk to the nurse. Child Life is consulted to talk with patient D about his understanding of his illness and how he has been feeling. Patient D makes a comment about how he, "Does what Mama asks." The legal team of the hospital becomes involved and patient D becomes closely monitored as Munchausen syndrome by proxy is suspected.

Case Study 3

The following fictional case study demonstrates Munchausen syndrome by proxy in which both the perpetrator and victim are adults.

Patient L is a 28-year-old woman who has been hospitalized for issues with her percutaneous endoscopic gastrostomy (PEG) tube. Patient L has a genetic disorder that puts her mental capacity to that of an 8-year-old. She had a PEG tube put in place last year owing to her inability to adequately absorb nutrition. She was brought in to the hospital by her 32-year-old sister, M. M has been her full-time caregiver for the past 7 years since the death of their mother.

Since being admitted, patient L has been complaining of nausea and vomiting. The treatment team have been unable to use her PEG tube owing to a blockage and there are plans to place another one. Her sister never leaves patient L's side and often speaks for her when communicating to the treatment team. At times, M gets very frustrated owing to the continuous nausea and vomiting that patient L experiences, which does not seem to improve.

The day before patient L is scheduled to get her new PEG tube, a nurse walks into her room. The curtain is closed so patient L and her sister did not see her enter. The nurse hears the sister tell patient L to take her medicine. When the nurse opens the curtain, she sees the sister spoon feeding something to patient L. The nurse asks what the sister is giving to patient L and she became very defensive. The medical team is asked to come in and talk with the sister because Munchausen syndrome by proxy is suspected.

SUMMARY

Through an understanding of diagnostic criteria, common characteristics, and treatment, clinicians can be better prepared to manage these syndromes when encountered. The case studies illustrated possible clinical scenarios of Munchausen syndrome and Munchausen syndrome by proxy. Both syndromes may be difficult to understand from a layman's perspective, because most individuals would have a hard time believing that a person would desire to make themselves seem to be sick or make a loved one seem to be sick. Nonetheless, these syndromes occur and require astute assessment skills. Developing and using an interdisciplinary team approach to include a legal representative is critical to expediting both diagnosis and treatment. Although these disorders are difficult to diagnosis, medical providers will be given ample opportunity, because the patient and/or their victims will be seeking medical attention for their symptoms. Therefore, it is important for health care providers to be knowledgeable of possible signs and symptoms of Munchausen syndrome and Munchausen syndrome by proxy to provide an early diagnosis. An early diagnosis supports the prevention and treatment of mental and physical consequences, which may ultimately lead to an untimely death.

REFERENCES

1. American Psychiatric Association. Diagnostic and statistical manual of mental disorders (DSM-5®). American Psychiatric Publishing; 2013.
2. Fliege H, Grimm A, Eckhardt-Henn A, et al. Frequency of ICD-10 factitious disorder: survey of senior hospital consultants and physicians in private practice. Psychosomatics 2007;48(1):60–4.
3. Sadock BJ, Sadock VA, Ruiz P, editors. Kaplan & Sadock's synopsis of psychiatry behavioral science/clinical psychiatry. Lippincott Williams & Wilkins; 2015.
4. Olry R, Haines DE. Historical and literary roots of Münchhausen syndromes: as intriguing as the syndromes themselves. Prog Brain Res 2012;206:123–41.
5. Yates GP, Feldman MD. Factitious disorder: a systematic review of 455 cases in the professional literature. Gen Hosp Psychiatry 2016;41:20–8.
6. Flaherty EG, MacMillan HL, Committee on Child Abuse and Neglect. Caregiver-fabricated illness in a child: a manifestation of child maltreatment. Pediatrics 2013;132(3):590–7.
7. Morrell B, Tilley DS. The role of nonperpetrating fathers in Munchausen syndrome by proxy: a review of the literature. J Pediatr Nurs 2012;27(4):328–35.
8. Bass C, Glaser D. Early recognition and management of fabricated or induced illness in children. Lancet 2014;383(9926):1412–21.
9. Marcus A, Ammermann C, Klein M, et al. Munchausen syndrome by proxy and factitious illness: symptomatology, parent-child interaction, and psychopathology of the parents. Eur Child Adolesc Psychiatry 1995;4(4):229–36.
10. Rand DC, Feldman MD. An explanatory model for Munchausen by proxy abuse. Int J Psychiatry Med 2001;31(2):113–26.
11. Beard KV. Protect the children: be on the lookout for Munchausen syndrome by proxy. RN 2007;70(12):33–6.
12. Sheridan MS. The deceit continues: an updated literature review of Munchausen syndrome by proxy. Child Abuse Negl 2003;27(4):431–51.
13. Meadow R. Munchausen syndrome by proxy abuse perpetrated by men. Arch Dis Child 1998;78(3):210–6.
14. Yates G, Bass C. The perpetrators of medical child abuse (Munchausen syndrome by proxy)–a systematic review of 796 cases. Child Abuse Negl 2017;72: 45–53.
15. Burton MC, Warren MB, Lapid MI, et al. Munchausen syndrome by adult proxy: a review of the literature. J Hosp Med 2015;10(1):32–5.
16. Squires JE, Squires RH. A review of Munchausen syndrome by proxy. Pediatr Ann 2013;42(4):e67–71.
17. Ali-Panzarella AZ, Bryant TJ, Marcovitch H, et al. Medical child abuse (Munchausen syndrome by proxy): multidisciplinary approach from a pediatric gastroenterology perspective. Curr Gastroenterol Rep 2017;19(4):14.
18. Galvin HK, Newton AW, Vandeven AM. Update on Munchausen syndrome by proxy. Curr Opin Pediatr 2005;17(2):252–7.
19. Greiner MV, Palusci VJ, Keeshin BR, et al. A preliminary screening instrument for early detection of medical child abuse. Hosp Pediatr 2013;3(1):39–44.

Evaluation and Treatment of Adrenal Dysfunction in the Primary Care Environment

Shannon Cole, DNP, APRN-BC

KEYWORDS

- Cushing's syndrome • Adrenocorticotropic hormone • Sympathetic nervous system
- Pheochromocytoma

KEY POINTS

- Adrenal Insufficiency is the clinical manifestation of deficient production or action of glucocorticoids or mineral corticoids.
- Adrenal Insufficiency is often disabling and occasionally lethal; however, it can be successfully treated if diagnosed early.
- Hypercortisolism, commonly called Cushing's Syndrome is caused by the overproduction of ACTH and consequent bilateral hyperplasia and overproduction of cortisol.
- The most common cause of Cushing's Syndrome is caused by prolonged exposure to glucocorticoids prescribed for inflammation.
- The primary care clinician should have knowledge related to the signs and symptoms, predisposing factors, diagnostic tests and treatment options for adrenal disorders.

INTRODUCTION

Adrenal dysfunction is an uncommon clinical disorder that occurs when there is interference with the normal functioning of the adrenal gland.[1–3] Adrenal disorders are classified by either hyperproduction or hypoproduction of cortisol and may be congenital or acquired. Adrenal insufficiency occurs when there is an inadequate level of basal or stress level cortisol. Conversely, Cushing's syndrome is characterized by an overproduction of adrenocorticotropic hormone (ACTH) with consequent bilateral adrenal hyperplasia and overproduction of cortisol.

The adrenal glands, located at the superior poles of the kidneys, produce hormones that regulate metabolism, the immune system, blood pressure, and other essential functions. Each gland is composed of 2 distinct parts, the adrenal medulla and the adrenal cortex. The adrenal medulla is regulated by the sympathetic nervous system and secretes the catecholamines, epinephrine, and norepinephrine. The adrenal cortex secretes 2 types of adrenocortical hormones, mineralocorticoids and glucocorticoids, along with a small amount of androgenic hormones. For the primary care clinician,

Vanderbilt University School of Nursing, 461 21st Avenue South, Nashville, TN 37240, USA
E-mail address: shannon.cole@vanderbilt.edu

Nurs Clin N Am 53 (2018) 385–394
https://doi.org/10.1016/j.cnur.2018.04.007   **nursing.theclinics.com**

the treatment of adrenal cortex disorders is more common; however, recognizing adrenal medullary dysfunction is also essential to ensure that patients are referred for appropriate specialty care.

ADRENAL MEDULLA

Disorders of the adrenal medulla arise primarily from neoplasms. Pheochromocytoma, the most common neoplasm, originates from chromaffin cells and excretes catecholamines. These neoplasms may also be of neural lineage, such as neuroblastomas and ganglioneuromas.[4,5] Fewer than 10% are malignant and the triad of symptoms include headache, diaphoresis, and palpitations. The classic sign is hypertension that is often refractory to treatment. In about 50% of patients, hypertension is sustained; however, some patients have relatively normal blood pressure with surges of elevations. Paroxysmal symptoms may vary from several times daily to weekly or monthly. The classic triad of symptoms include headache, diaphoresis, and palpitations. Less common symptoms include anxiety, pain in the chest or abdomen, fatigue, and weight loss. Given the life-threatening nature of labile hypertension, a high index of suspicion is imperative. Typically, pheochromocytoma is diagnosed with evidence of catecholamines or their metabolites in the urine. After a positive urine test a computed tomography scan, MRI, or ultrasound examination (when radiation must be minimized in pregnancy, infants, and children) may be used to visualize a tumor.

Diseases of the adrenal medulla are fortunately rare; however, they are potentially life threatening. The primary care clinician must be able to recognize the signs and symptoms of adrenal medullar dysfunction. Proper treatment is managed by endocrinology, surgery, and oncology (for the <10% of cases that are malignant).

ADRENAL CORTEX

The adrenal cortex, the outer layer of the adrenal gland, is composed of 3 distinct zones and is responsible for the production of vital hormones, cortisol and aldosterone. The outer zone, the zona glomerulosa, produces the mineralocorticoid aldosterone, which is responsible for sodium reabsorption and potassium excretion, which regulates extracellular fluid volume and arterial blood pressure. Dysfunction of the zona glomerulosa may result in death owing to retention of high levels of potassium and excess loss of sodium.[6] The zona fasciculata and the zona reticularis produce glucocorticoids. Cortisol, the most important glucocorticoid, regulates metabolism and mediates the response to stress. It is essential when the body experiences stress such as with surgery, trauma, or serious infection. Without proper amounts of cortisol, the body is unable to cope with major stress, which can lead to crisis and death. **Table 1** lists the adrenal hormones and their potencies secreted by the adrenal cortex.

ADRENAL INSUFFICIENCY

Adrenal insufficiency is the clinical manifestation of deficient production or action of glucocorticoids and/or mineralocorticoids. It is a potentially life-threatening disorder that can result from primary adrenal failure or secondary adrenal disease owing to impairment of the hypothalamic–pituitary axis.[7–10] Although often disabling and occasionally lethal, adrenal insufficiency can be treated successfully if diagnosed early. The primary care clinician should have knowledge related to signs and symptoms, predisposing factors, diagnostic tests, and treatment modalities. **Box 1** lists symptoms, clinical signs, and laboratory results associated with adrenal insufficiency.

Table 1	
Adrenal hormones	
Type	**Potency**
Mineralocorticoids	
Aldosterone	Very potent: Accounts for about 90% of all mineralocorticoid activity
Desoxycortisone	Weak: 1/15th as potent as aldosterone
Cortisol	Weak: 80× is excreted with only slight mineralocorticoid activity.
Glucocorticoids	
Cortisol	Very potent: Accounts for 95% of all glucocorticoid activity
Corticosterone	Weak: Accounts for 4% of total glucocorticoid activity

From Guyton AC, Hall J. Textbook of medical physiology. Philadelphia: W.B. Saunders; 1996; with permission.

The cardinal clinical symptoms of adrenal insufficiency were first described by Thomas Addison in 1855.[11] These include weakness, fatigue, anorexia, abdominal pain, orthostatic hypotension, salt craving, and hyperpigmentation of the skin. Severe symptoms warrant emergency medical intervention and are characterized by severe hypotensive crisis, and a clouded sensorium with severe musculoskeletal and abdominal pain, along with fever.

Adrenal insufficiency is characterized by the inability of the adrenal cortex to produce sufficient amounts of glucocorticoids and/or mineralocorticoids. It is classified as primary, secondary, or tertiary. **Table 2** lists the 3 types of adrenal insufficiencies, common causes, and physiologic effects. Glucocorticoids are essential for maintaining vascular tone, blood pressure, cardiac function, and normalization of glucose. Mineralocorticoids are responsible for the regulation of serum sodium and potassium concentrations and are essential for maintain vascular volume.[12–15]

Primary adrenal insufficiency (PAI) occurs as a result of the destruction of the adrenal cortex. Its most common cause is autoimmune injury in developed countries and

---

Box 1
Symptoms, clinical signs and laboratory results associated with adrenal insufficiency

Symptoms
- Fatigue
- Loss of appetite
- Salt craving
- Nausea, vomiting, diarrhea, abdominal pain
- Dizziness
- Musculoskeletal pain
- Collapse

Signs
- Hyperpigmentation of skin
- Weight loss
- Hypotension
- Shock

Laboratory Results
- Hyponatremia
- Hyperkalemia
- Hypoglycemia

Data from Burton C, Cottrell E, Edwards J. Addison's disease: identification and management in primary care. Br J Gen Pract 2015;65(638):488–90.

Table 2
Types of adrenal insufficiency

Type	Common Cause	Effect
Primary	Autoimmune injury	Destruction of the adrenal cortex
Secondary	Prolonged treatment with systemic or inhaled steroids	Disruption of the ability to make steroids
Tertiary	Tumor invasion, radiation, stroke or infection	Inadequate corticotropin-releasing hormone from the hypothalamus

infection in developing countries.[16,17] Adrenal injury may also occur due to hemorrhage as seen with meningococcemia or secondary to infarction.

Secondary or central adrenal insufficiency represents a potentially life-threatening disorder that results from reduced cortisol production secondary to impaired production of ACTH produced by the pituitary gland. ACTH stimulates the production of steroids and, without it, steroid production is halted.[18] Secondary adrenal insufficiency may arise with prolonged exposure to systemic or high-dose inhaled steroids or from pituitary disease that impede the release of ACTH, as seen with adenomas or craniopharyngiomas[16]

Tertiary adrenal insufficiency is caused by impaired synthesis of corticotropin-releasing hormone, which leads to ACTH deficiency.[18] This can occur with tumor invasion, stroke, or infection. Prolonged deficiency may lead to adrenal atrophy.

Diagnostics

Adrenal insufficiency may be difficult to diagnose. Tests that measure cortisol and aldosterone will be used to make a definitive diagnosis. The ACTH stimulation test is the most specific diagnostic test, and it considered the gold standard for assessing the adrenal glands response to stress. For this test, cortisol levels are measured before and after a synthetic form of ACTH is administered by injection. The standard dose is 250 μg for adults and children 2 years of age and older, 125 μg for children less than 2, and 15 μg/kg for infants. In healthy individuals, the cortisol should double from a baseline of 20 to 30 μg/dL.

An insulin-induced hypoglycemia test may also be used to determine how the hypothalamus, pituitary, and adrenal glands respond to stress. For this test, glucose and cortisol levels are measured before an injection of 0.15 U/kg of body weight of fast-acting regular insulin, and again at 30, 45, and 90 minutes.[19–21] In patients thought to have hypopituitarism or PAI, the insulin dose is decreased to 0.1 U/kg of body weight and for patients who are obese and/or have diabetes, the dose is increased to 0.25 U/kg of body weight. This test is potentially dangerous and is done under direct medical supervision in the hospital setting. Intravenous glucose should be available because severe hypoglycemia may occur. It is not recommended for the elderly or for patients who have evidence of myocardial disease or a history of seizures.

Treatment

Adrenal crisis can be fatal. In patients with persistent vomiting, muscle weakness, dehydration, hypotension, headache, and extreme fatigue, hospital admission is necessary because this is a medical emergency. For patients who exhibit symptoms and seem to be stable, assessing a basic metabolic profile along with a cortisol stimulation test will lead to proper diagnosis.

Lifelong oral steroid medications are usually indicated and adjusted by an endocrinologist. Both glucocorticoids (hydrocortisone) and mineralocorticoids (fludrocortisone), and often an increase of sodium chloride to compensate for increased renal loss, are prescribed. Replacement therapy should mimic the endogenous cortisol rhythm and be at the lowest dose that alleviates symptoms and avoids glucocorticoid excess. Additionally, education on how illness and/or injury necessitate an increase in glucocorticoid/mineralocorticoid dosages will be addressed with patients.[22,23] **Box 2** lists common synthetic adrenal hormones that may be prescribed as treatment for severe adrenal insufficiency and adrenal crisis.

PRIMARY ADRENAL INSUFFICIENCY IN CHILDREN

PAI in children arises from abnormalities in the development of the adrenal gland, impaired steroidogenesis, resistance to ACTH, action or adrenal destruction. Most cases of PAI in childhood are inherited and monogenic in origin and caused by disruption of hormone productions causing congenital adrenal hyperplasia (CAH). CAH occurs 1 in 10,000 to 18,000 births and is responsible for most cases of PAI in children.[24] CAH is an autosomal recessive disorder associated with deficiency of the enzymes necessary for cortisol biosynthesis. This deficiency increases ACTH production that leads to hyperplasia and an accumulation of precursor steroids that are diverted to androgens.

The clinical presentation of CAH may be mild or severe based on the degree of enzyme impairment. The most common signs and symptoms are anorexia, weight loss, fatigue, myalgia, joint pain, hypotension, hyponatremia, hypoglycemia, lymphocytosis, and eosinophilia. Signs may include hyperpigmentation of skin, nail beds, mucous membranes, and palmar creases. Newborns often exhibit hyperbilirubinemia and infants may experience failure to thrive and undervirilization owing to excess androgens causing genital ambiguity.[24]

Treatment of CAH includes replacement of the glucocorticoids and mineralocorticoids, mainly hydrocortisone and fludrocortisone. For adrenal crisis, intravenous fluids and salt replacement is necessary. Primary treatment goals include maintaining electrolyte balance and attaining normal physical growth and pubertal development. It is crucial to maintain normal cortisol excretion, because excessive treatment may lead to growth suppression, obesity, the metabolic syndrome, and osteoporosis. **Box 3** lists common signs and symptoms, laboratory findings, and treatments for children presenting with adrenal insufficiency.

CUSHING'S SYNDROME

Harvey Cushing first described a patient with hypercortisolism in 1912. The patient presented with rapidly acquired central obesity, hypertrichosis, amenorrhea, and muscle weakness. The physical examination revealed a round face, and supraclavicular and posterior cervical fat pads; it was noted that the skin was dry with

---

Box 2
Synthetic adrenal hormones

Mineralocorticoids
- 9α-Fluorocortisol: Weak (slightly more potent than cortisol)
- Cortisone: Weak (slightly more potent than cortisol)

Glucocorticoids
- Prednisone: Very potent (4× more than cortisol)
- Methylprednisone: Very potent (5× more than cortisol)
- Dexamethasone: Very potent (30× more than cortisol)

> **Box 3**
> **Adrenal insufficiency in children**
>
> Symptoms
> - Anorexia
> - Weight loss
> - Fatigue
> - Muscle and joint pain
>
> Signs
> - Hyperpigmentation of skin, nail beds and mucous membranes
> - Palmar creases
> - Ambiguous genitalia (infants)
> - Hypotension
>
> Abnormal Laboratory tests
> - Hyponatremia
> - Hyperglycemia
> - Lymphocytosis
> - Eosinophilia
> - Hyperbilirubinemia (infants)
>
> Treatment
> - Replacement of glucocorticoids/mineralocorticoids
> - Intravenous fluids (adrenal crisis)
> - Sodium replacement (adrenal crisis)
> - Attaining normal growth and development

considerable pigmentation with multiple ecchymoses and striae. Cushing syndrome, a rare disease that results from prolonged exposure to high circulating levels of cortisol can be challenging to identify and treat. Although some clinical presentations are straightforward, such as the patient first described by Harvey Cushing, most are often highly variable.[25,26]

Hypercortisolism, commonly called Cushing's syndrome is caused by the overproduction of ACTH with consequent bilateral adrenal hyperplasia and overproduction of cortisol. There are 2 main etiologies: endogenous hypercortisolism and exogenous hypercortisolism. Exogenous hypercortisolism, the most common cause of Cushing's syndrome, is mostly iatrogenic and is caused by prolonged use of corticosteroids. The endogenous type results from excessive production or adrenal gland cortisol production and can be ACTH dependent or ACTH independent.[25] Cushing's disease accounts for 80% of endogenous hypercortisolism and is caused by ACTH-dependent cortisol excess owing to a pituitary adenoma.[27]

The most common cause of Cushing's syndrome (exogenous or iatrogenic) is caused by prolonged exposure of glucocorticoids prescribed for chronic inflammation and treatment of autoimmune and neoplastic disorders. Although the oral route is most commonly associated with exogenous Cushing's syndrome, any mode of delivery, including inhaled, topical, or injectable, may be contributory.[25] Treatment for iatrogenic Cushing's syndrome involves tapering off glucocorticoids slowly.

Symptoms of Cushing's Syndrome in adults are weight gain (especially in the trunk, and often not accompanied by weight gain in the arms and legs), hypertension, and changes in mood, memory, and concentration. Additional problems such as muscle weakness may arise secondary to loss of protein. A comprehensive list includes:

- Weight gain,
- Hypertension,
- Short-term memory loss,

- Irritability,
- Excessive hair growth (women),
- Red face,
- Extra fat around the neck,
- Round face,
- Fatigue,
- Easy bruising,
- Depression,
- Weakened bones,
- Acne,
- Baldness (women),
- Edema to feet/legs, and
- Hyperglycemia.[27]

Diagnosis

After a thorough drug history, excluding excessive exogenous glucocorticoid exposure,[27] recommends against widespread testing for Cushing's syndrome and instead suggests testing for Cushing's syndrome in the following groups:

- Patients with unusual features for age, such as osteoporosis and hypertension;
- Patients with multiple and progressive features, particularly those that are more predictive of Cushing's syndrome;
- Children with decreasing height percentile and increasing weight; and
- Patients with adrenal incidentaloma compatible with adenoma.

For initial testing,[27] the following tests are recommended based on the suitability for a given patient:

- Urine free cortisol on at least 2 occasions;
- Late-night salivary cortisol (2 measurements),
- 1 mg dexamethasone suppression test; and
- Longer low-dose dexamethasone suppression test (2 mg/d for 48 hours).

For individuals with normal test results who have clinical features suggestive of Cushing's disease and adrenal incidentaloma or suspected cyclic hypercortisolism, the recommendation is for further evaluation by an endocrinologist. For individuals with normal test results where Cushing's syndrome is unlikely, reevaluation in 6 months is suggested if signs and/or symptoms persist. Last, individuals with at least 1 abnormal result should have an endocrinology consult to confirm or exclude the diagnosis.

Treatment of Cushing's Syndrome

The Endocrine Society's Clinical Practice Guideline (2015) suggests normalizing cortisol levels or action of its receptors to eliminate the signs and symptoms along with treating comorbidities associated with hypercortisolism.[28] We recommended avoiding treatment designed to normalize cortisol or its action when there is:

- Not an established diagnosis of Cushing's syndrome; and
- Only borderline biochemical abnormality of the hypothalamic–pituitary axis without specific signs of Cushing's syndrome.

The optimal adjunctive management includes the following:

- Provide education to patients and families about the disease, treatment options and what is to be expected with remission.

- A multidisciplinary team, including an endocrinologist, should take patients values and preferences into consideration while providing treatment options to the patient.
- Patients should be evaluated for risk factors such as venous thrombosis.
- Clinicians should discuss and offer age-appropriate vaccinations, particularly influenza, herpes zoster, and pneumococcal.
- All patients should receive monitoring and adjuvant treatment for cortisol-dependent comorbidities, including:
  o Psychiatric disorders,
  o Diabetes,
  o Hypertension,
  o Hypokalemia,
  o Infections,
  o Dyslipidemia,
  o Osteoporosis, and
  o Poor physical fitness.

First-line treatment options for Cushing's disease involve resection of the primary lesion (cancer, adenoma, or bilateral disease). For patients who underwent a noncurative surgery or for whom surgery was not possible, a shared decision making approach is suggested because there are second-line therapies (repeat resection, radiotherapy, medical therapy, and adrenalectomy).

Early detection and treatment is necessary to decrease the high morbidity and mortality associated with Cushing's syndrome. Cushing's syndrome is rare; however, the effects may be devastating. For patients with Cushing's syndrome caused by exogenous hypercortisolism, tapering glucocorticoid medications is the most effective treatment. Endogenous hypercortisolism often requires surgery, which may not be curative.

SUMMARY

Adrenal insufficiency (Addison's disease) and Cushing's syndrome are rare disorders characterized by abnormal secretion of adrenal hormones.[29] All patients with adrenal insufficiency and many with Cushing's syndrome require life-long therapy that has the potential to impact the quality of life of patients dramatically both physically and emotionally. Adrenal disorder management requires patients and families to gain a significant amount of knowledge related to treatment, self-care and how to react quickly in critical situations. Knowledge deficits related to management of an adrenal crisis may cause patients to become critically ill and may even cause death. Ongoing patient/family teaching is crucial for proper disease management and for sustaining the quality of life for patients diagnosed with adrenal dysfunction.

The primary care clinician is responsible for recognizing the signs and symptoms of adrenal dysfunction. Often these can be subtle; however, adrenal dysfunction should be listed as a possible differential diagnosis for patients who present with the following sign, symptoms, and laboratory results.

Adrenal Insufficiency
- Weakness
- Fatigue
- Anorexia
- Abdominal pain
- Orthostatic hypotension

- Salt craving
- Hyperpigmentation of the skin
- Hyponatremia
- Hyperkalemia
- Hypoglycemia

Cushing's Syndrome
- Weight gain
- Hypertension
- Irritability
- Red face
- Extra neck fat
- Easy bruising
- Short-term memory loss
- Edema to feet/legs
- Hyperglycemia

In most cases, adrenal disorders are managed by endocrinologists; however, it is the role of the primary clinician to recognize the symptoms, perform a thorough history, physical examination, laboratory evaluation, and in some cases a computed tomography scan or MRI. Once the patient has been properly diagnosed, the primary clinician and endocrinologist should work as a team to maximize optimal treatment and maximization of patient outcomes and quality of life.

REFERENCES

1. Artalejo AR, Olivos-Ore LA. Alpha2-adrenoreceptors in adrenomedullary chromaffin cells: functional role and pathophysiological implications. Pflugers Arch 2018;470:61–6.
2. Bonnet-Serrano F, Bertherat J. Genetics of tumors of the adrenal cortex. Endocr Relat Cancer 2017;25:R131–52.
3. Bornstein SR. Predisposing factors for adrenal insufficiency. N Engl J Med 2009; 360(22):2328–39.
4. Fung MM, Viveros OH, O'Connor DT. Diseases of the adrenal medulla. Acta Physiol (Oxf) 2008;192(2):325–35.
5. Glenn JA, Kiernan CM, Yen TW, et al. Management of suspected adrenal metastases at 2 academic medical centers. Am J Surg 2016;(211):664–70.
6. Pignatti EI, Sining L, Carlone DL, et al. Regulation of zonation and homeostasis in the adrenal cortex. Mol Cell Endocrinol 2016;441:146–55.
7. Charmandari E, Nicolaides NC, Chrousos GP. Adrenal insufficiency. Lancet 2014; 6736(13):61684–700.
8. de Diego MA, Gandai L, Garcia AG. A physiologic view of the central and peripheral mechanisms that regulate the release of catecholamines at the adrenal medulla. Acta Physiol (Oxf) 2008;192(22):287–301.
9. Dorin RI, Qualls CR, Crapo LM. Diagnosis of adrenal insufficiency. Ann Intern Med 2003;(139):194–204.
10. El-Maouche D, Wiebke AP, Merke DP. Congenital adrenal hyperplasia. Lancet 2017;390(10108):2194–210.
11. Puar HK, Stikkelbroek MM, Smans CC, et al. Adrenal crisis: still a deadly event in the 21st century. Am J Med 2016;129(3):339.e1-9.
12. Kola B, Grossman AB. Dynamic testing in Cushing's syndrome. Pituitary 2008;11: 155–62.

13. Lymperopoulos A, Brill A, McCrink AK. GPCRs of adrenal chromaffin cells & catecholamines: the plot thickens. Int J Cell Biol 2016;77(Pt-B):213–9.

14. Moloney S, Dowling M. Early intervention and management of adrenal insufficiency in children. Nurs Child Young People 2012;7:25–8.

15. Nieman LK. Insulin induced hypoglycemia test, 5 July 2017. Available at: https://uptodate.com/contents/insulin-induced-hypoglycemia-test. Accessed January 10, 2018.

16. Hittle K, Hsieh S, Sheeran P. Acute adrenal crisis masquerading as septic shock in a healthy young woman. J Pediatr Health Care 2010;24(1):48–52.

17. Hong AR, Ryu OH, Kim SY, et al. Characteristics of Korean Patients with primary adrenal insufficiency: a registry-based nationwide survey in Korea. Endocrinol Metab 2017;32:466–74.

18. Paragliola RM, Corsello SM. Secondary adrenal insufficiency: from the physiopathology to the possible role of modified-release hydrocortisone treatment. Minerva Endocrinol 2018;43(2):183–97.

19. Bornstein SR, Allolio B, Arit W, et al. Diagnosis and treatment of primary adrenal insufficiency: an endocrine society clinical practice guideline. J Clin Endocrinol Metab 2016;101(2):364–89.

20. Boscaro M, Arnaldi G. Approach to the patient with possible Cushing's syndrome. J Clin Endocrinol Metab 2009;94(9):3121–31.

21. Carey RM. Adrenal disease update 2011. J Clin Endocrinol Metab 2011;96(12):3583–91.

22. Husebye ES, Allolio B, Arit W, et al. Consensus statement on the diagnosis, treatment and follow-up of patients with primary adrenal insufficiency. J Intern Med 2014;275(2):104–15.

23. Kanczkowski W, Mariko S, Bornstein SR. The adrenal gland microenvironment in health, disease and during regeneration. Hormones 2017;16(3):251–65.

24. Guran T. Latest insights on the etiology and management of primary adrenal insufficiency in children. J Clin Res Pediatr Endocrinol 2017;9(2):9–22.

25. Sharma ST, Nieman LK, Feelders RA. Cushing's syndrome: epidemiology and developments in disease management. Clin Epidemiol 2015;7:281–93.

26. Vance ML. Treatment of patients with a pituitary adenoma: one clinician's experience. Neurosurg Focus 2004;16(4):1–6.

27. Nieman LK, Biller K, Finding JW, et al. The diagnosis of Cushing's syndrome: an endocrine society clinical practice guideline. J Clin Endocrinol Metab 2008;93(5):1526–40.

28. Nieman LK, Biller MK, Findling JW, et al. Treatment of Cushing's syndrome: an endocrine society clinical practice guideline. J Clin Endocrinol Metab 2015;100(8):2807–31.

29. Kauw D, Repping-Wuts H, Noordzij A, et al. The contribution of online peer-to-peer communication among patients with adrenal disease to patient-centered care. J Med Internet Res 2015;17(2):e54.

Male and Female Hypogonadism

Angela Richard-Eaglin, DNP, MSN, APRN, FNP-BC

KEYWORDS

- Hypogonadism • Kallmann syndrome • Turner syndrome
- Hypergonadotropic hypogonadism • Testosterone replacement therapy
- Hypogonadism treatment • Hypogonadotropic hypogonadism
- Klinefelter syndrome

KEY POINTS

- Primary hypogonadism is caused by gonadal (testicular or ovarian) failure.
- Secondary hypogonadism is the result of a dysfunction at any level within the hypothalamus and/or pituitary.
- Clinical presentation and clinical management are based on age of onset, signs and symptoms, and laboratory/diagnostic test results.

BACKGROUND

Hypogonadism refers to a clinical syndrome caused by a disruption of any level of the hypothalamic–pituitary–gonadal axis.[1–5] It is classified as primary or secondary, based on the cause. Primary hypogonadism, also known as hypergonadotropic hypogonadism, occurs as a result of a dysfunction of the gonads (testes in men and ovaries in women).[1–6] Hypogonadism is caused by several factors, including: genetic and developmental disorders, infection, kidney disease, liver disease, autoimmune disorders, chemotherapy, radiation, surgery, and trauma.[1–6] Preexisting autoimmune disorders increase the risk of autoimmune-related damage to the gonads.[6] Hypogonadotropic hypogonadism or secondary hypogonadism results from dysfunction of the hypothalamus and/or the pituitary gland.[1–3] Secondary hypogonadism is mainly characterized by isolated gonadotropin-releasing hormone (GnRH) deficiency.[1–6]

Kallmann syndrome is the most common genetic cause of hypogonadotropic hypogonadism in men and women and is associated with anosmia or hyposmia.[1–8] In addition, patients with Kallmann syndrome may also have cleft lip and palate and other

Disclosure Statement: The author does not have any relationship with a commercial company that has a direct financial interest in subject matter or materials discussed in article or with a company making a competing product.
Healthcare in Adult Populations Division, Duke University School of Nursing, DUMC 3322, 307 Trent Drive, Durham, NC 27710, USA
E-mail address: angela.richard-eaglin@duke.edu

craniofacial defects, neurosensory deafness, digital anomalies, unilateral renal agenesis, and other neurologic defects.[5] Other causes of secondary hypogonadism include morbid obesity, medications (ie, glucocorticoids, opioids), pituitary disorders (including tumors or damage), eating disorders, anabolic steroid abuse, hyperprolactinemia, aging, or may be idiopathic.[1–3,5]

In both men and women patients presenting with delayed puberty, it is important to differentiate between constitutional delay of puberty and hypogonadism, as constitutional delay is much more common.[4] Obtaining a careful and comprehensive health history that includes signs and symptoms, medication history, activity level, eating patterns, and family history is vital. A complete physical examination is also warranted to aid in the diagnosis of hypogonadism. In the absence of specific signs and symptoms to direct the workup for suspected hypogonadism, other conditions, such as acute infection, autoimmune disorders, and thyroid dysfunction, with a similar clinical presentation must be excluded.[4] The following tests are helpful in differentiating hypogonadism from other conditions: a complete white blood count, a sedimentation rate, a comprehensive metabolic panel, a celiac screening, thyroid function tests, and a urinalysis.[4]

Treatment for primary and secondary hypogonadism for men and women involves replacement of sex steroids to initiate development and maintenance of secondary sex characteristics.[4,5] Sex steroid replacement does not induce fertility in men or women.[4,5] Gonadotropin or GnRH replacement is prescribed when fertility is desired.[4,5] When hypogonadism is a result of a pituitary or hypothalamic disorder, surgery and radiation therapy may be indicated.[4]

MALE HYPOGONADISM

Male hypogonadism refers to a clinical syndrome that occurs when the testes fail to produce physiologic levels of testosterone, normal sperm levels, or both. Primary hypogonadism, also known as testicular hypogonadism in men, is a result of testicular dysfunction. It is associated with low serum testosterone levels, spermatogenesis impairment, and increased levels of the gonadotropins, luteinizing hormone (LH), and follicle-stimulating hormone (FSH).[1–6] Male hypergonadotropic hypogonadism (primary hypogonadism) is most commonly caused by Klinefelter syndrome, unilateral or bilateral cryptorchidism, mumps orchitis, radiation and chemotherapy, medications (ie, glucocorticoids and ketoconazole), testicular torsion, and trauma.[1–5] Hypogonadotropic hypogonadism or secondary hypogonadism results from disorders of the hypothalamus and the pituitary gland, causing low serum testosterone levels, decreased spermatogenesis, and low or inappropriately normal levels of LH and FSH.[1–3]

Diagnosis

The diagnosis of male hypogonadism is based on signs and symptoms in combination with serum testosterone levels. The clinical presentation of men with hypogonadism is consistent with the age of onset.[1] Clinicians should begin the diagnostic workup by obtaining a comprehensive health history, which should include questions regarding the following: existing systemic medical conditions, family medical history, drug use or misuse, eating habits (to ascertain presence of eating disorders), exercise practices, and prescription medications. The signs and symptoms are variable and modified by age of onset, duration and severity of hormone deficiency, individual androgen deficiency and sensitivity, comorbidities, and history of previous testosterone therapy.[1–3] Clinical manifestations of hypogonadism in prepubertal men include delayed or incomplete sexual development, eunuchoidism, high-pitched voice, sparse body hair, poorly developed skeletal muscles, micropenis, and delayed epiphyseal closure.[1–3,5,6] Postpubertal clinical manifestations in men include hot flashes, decreased libido, erectile dysfunction, decreased scrotal size, body hair loss, muscle atrophy and decreased strength, fatigue, gynecomastia, prolactinoma, irritability, depression, and sleep disturbance.[1–6]

During periods of acute illness recovery, men often have transient hypogonadotropic hypogonadism, which improves as the illness is resolved.[3] For this reason, the diagnostic workup should be deferred until such time that acute conditions are resolved. Conversely, there are certain conditions that increase the prevalence of low testosterone and induce symptoms such as sexual dysfunction, weight loss, and weakness, which warrant evaluation of serum testosterone levels. These conditions include type 2 diabetes, end-stage renal disease, and chronic obstructive pulmonary disease.[1–3] Men with conditions such as human immunodeficiency virus (HIV)–related weight loss, a pituitary mass, law trauma fractures, or treatment with glucocorticoids or opioids may also warrant evaluation of serum testosterone levels, irrespective of symptoms.[1–3]

A reliable assay must be used to measure at least 2 morning serum testosterone levels on a minimum of 2 occasions.[1–3] If the total testosterone level is less than 9 to 12 nmol/L (250–350 ng/dL), a free testosterone may be measured and a serum LH and FSH should be ordered (**Fig. 1**).[1–3] A diagnosis of primary hypogonadism should be suspected if the serum testosterone level and the LH and FSH levels are elevated. If LH and FSH levels are low or inappropriately normal, secondary hypogonadism is the suspected diagnosis.[1–3] After these results are obtained, further symptom-directed testing is warranted to identify the underlying cause and guide treatment (see **Fig. 1**).[1–3] Obtain a karyotype to rule out Klinefelter syndrome in men with primary hypogonadism of unknown cause, especially if the testicular volume is less than 6 mL.[1–3] A minimum of 2 seminal analyses should be obtained in men being evaluated for infertility.[1]

If secondary hypogonadism is diagnosed, further diagnostic screening may be warranted to exclude pituitary neoplasia, infiltrative diseases (ie, hemochromatosis), obstructive sleep apnea, and genetic disorders that contribute to hypogonadism.[1] Patients with hypogonadotropic hypogonadism are examined for dysmorphic features, such as short stature, polydactyly, anosmia (ie, Kallmann syndrome), and extreme obesity (ie, Prader-Willi syndrome).[1] Once other causes of secondary hypogonadism have been ruled out, a diagnosis of idiopathic hypogonadotropic hypogonadism is made.[1,5]

Prognosis

Morbidity for men with hypogonadism includes decreased quality of life related to sexual health, infertility, and an increased risk of osteoporosis.[6] There is no known increase in mortality related to hypogonadism.[1,6] Although it is a chronic condition that cannot be cured, it is treatable.[6]

Screening

The impact of hypogonadism on mortality, long-term benefits and effects of testosterone therapy, and the long-term consequences on low testosterone levels have yet to be determined. There is also no clinical trial evidence of the predictive value or cost-effectiveness of generalized screening of the male population for hypogonadism. Therefore, routine screening for hypogonadism in the general male population cannot be justified.[1,2,7]

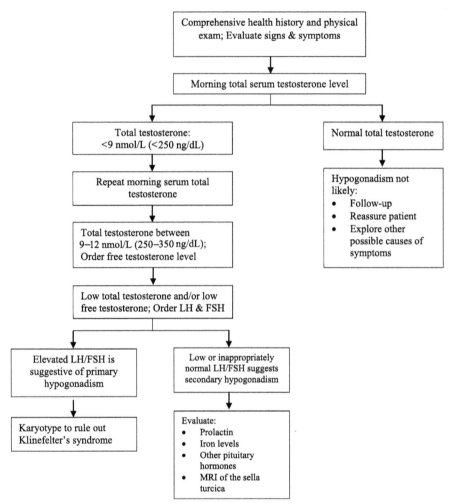

Fig. 1. Diagnostic workup for male hypogonadism. A comprehensive health history should be obtained at the initial visit to determine existence of systemic disorders, substance use/abuse (opioids, glucocorticoids, anabolic steroids), and eating habits (signs and symptoms of anorexia nervosa). Testosterone reference ranges vary by laboratory; therefore, providers should use the ranges provided by the laboratory in their clinical practice. Prolactin levels guide diagnosis of prolactinoma. MRI should be ordered on a case-by-case basis and directly related to the patient's clinical presentation. (*Data from* Bhasin S, Cunningham GR, Hayes FJ, et al. Testosterone therapy in men with androgen defieciency syndromes: an endocrine society clinical practice guideline. J Clin Endocrinol Metab 2010;95(6):2536–59.)

Clinical Management

The goal of treatment of hypogonadism is to restore sexual function and well-being, induce and/or maintain secondary sex characteristics, restore fertility, and improve bone mineral density, and muscle mass.[1,4,5] Testosterone therapy is contraindicated and should not be initiated in men with a history of breast or prostate cancer, men with a hematocrit greater than 50%, untreated severe obstructive sleep apnea, poorly controlled heart failure, and men with severe lower urinary tract infection.[1–3] Prostate cancer risk should be assessed before initiation of testosterone therapy. Men with the following conditions should not receive testosterone therapy without evaluation by a urologist: a palpable prostate induration or nodule, prostate-specific antigen (PSA) greater than 4 ng/mL in non–high-risk men, or a PSA greater than 3 ng/mL in men at high risk for prostate cancer (ie, African American men and men with a first-degree relative with a history of prostate cancer).[1,2,5] The goal of testosterone treatment is to induce serum testosterone levels to mid-normal range in healthy young men (**Table 1**).[1] The Endocrine Society recommends that testosterone therapy should

Table 1
Hypogonadism management in men: US-approved testosterone therapy

	Route	Dosing	Testosterone Level Monitoring	Patient Education
Injectable preparations Long-acting testosterone esters: • Testosterone enanthate or cypionate	Intramuscular	For pubertal induction: 50–75 mg/mo; gradually increase every 6 mo to 100–150 mg/mo Adult men: 75–100 mg weekly or 150–200 mg biweekly	3–6 mo after initiation of therapy, then yearly 3–6 mo after initiation of therapy, then yearly	Advise patient that changes in mood may occur
Transdermal preparations • Testosterone patch • Testosterone gel 1%	Transdermal Transdermal	5–10 mg patch applied daily 5–10 g of gel containing 50–100 mg of testosterone, applied daily	3–12 h after application Any time of day after 1 wk of treatment	Apply to skin of upper arm, back, or thigh in nonpressure location. A skin reaction may occur at the site of application. Advise patient to cover application site with a shirt; testosterone can be transferred through skin to skin contact; wash skin with soap and water before skin contact with others; leave gel on for at least 4–6 h before washing
Buccal testosterone tablets	Buccal	30 mg controlled release bioadhesive tablets twice daily (every 12 h)	Immediately before or after application	Advise patient that taste alterations and irritation to gums and oral mucosa may occur
2% Axillary testosterone solution[3]	Axilla[3]	60–120 mg topical solution in axillae daily[3]	2–8 h after application[3]	Skin irritation may occur[3]

Data from Refs.[1–3,5]

not be offered to all older men with low testosterone levels, but rather should be offered to older men on a symptom-related case-by-case basis.[1]

Monitoring of Testosterone Therapy

Serum testosterone levels should be monitored at specific points in time after initiation of testosterone therapy (see **Table 1**). A hematocrit should be checked at baseline, at 3 to 6 months, and then yearly.[1,2] Therapy should be discontinued if the hematocrit is greater than 54% and should remain discontinued until the hematocrit returns to normal.[1] Patients with an elevated hematocrit should be assessed for hypoxia and sleep apnea.[1] Once the hematocrit returns to normal, testosterone therapy should be restarted at a decreased dose.[1] In men aged 40 years and older with a baseline PSA greater than 0.6 ng/mL, a PSA level and digital rectal examination should be performed before initiating treatment and then at 3 to 6 months after starting treatment.[1,2] A urology consult is recommended for a PSA greater than 1.4 ng/mL in a 12-month period of receiving testosterone treatment or in the event of an abnormal digital rectal examination.[1] Hypogonadal men with osteoporosis or low trauma fracture should have a bone mineral density test of the lumbar spine and/or the femoral neck after 1 to 2 years of testosterone therapy.[1]

Controversies and Evidence

Hypogonadism (testosterone deficiency) contributes to many health problems in men, yet many providers remain reluctant to prescribe testosterone replacement therapy due to concern regarding the possible adverse effects.[8] However, there is recent research evidence refuting the findings from previous studies that suggest that testosterone therapy increases cardiovascular risk, stroke incidence, and prostate cancer incidence.[8–20] Traish states that previous clinical trials regarding the association of prostate cancer with testosterone therapy, such as the Reduction by Dutasteride of Prostate Cancer Events (REDUCE) trial and others, did not show an association between prostate cancer risk and testosterone therapy.[8]

Morgentaler and colleagues[12] analyzed some of the previous cardiovascular risk related to testosterone therapy studies and found that the findings were not reliable or credible based on contaminated data, flaws in the methodology, and use of nonvalidated statistical methods.[9,13] Traish also suggests that data from studies reporting an increased risk in cardiovascular events in men treated with testosterone therapy must be viewed cautiously based on the flaws in the methodology of those studies.[8] In a real-life observational study on long-term testosterone use in men with hypogonadism and cardiovascular effects, Traish and colleagues[9] found that cardiovascular mortality was significantly reduced in the testosterone therapy group. Because of the negative effects of testosterone deficiency in men, including decreased quality of life, decreased musculature and strength, and the decreased glycometabolic and cardiometabolic function, testosterone replacement therapy to normalize testosterone levels to improve overall health in men with hypogonadism is recommended.[8,9] The Endocrine Society clinical practice guidelines recommend testosterone therapy to promote bone health for men with low testosterone levels who are also receiving high doses of glucocorticoids.[1] The guidelines also recommend testosterone replacement therapy to maintain lean bone mass and muscle strength in HIV-infected men with low testosterone levels.

FEMALE HYPOGONADISM

Female hypogonadism refers to a clinical syndrome that occurs as a result of ovarian failure, causing the ovaries to produce less than physiologic levels of estrogen.[4,5] The most common clinical feature in prepubertal women with hypogonadism is delayed pubertal onset or primary amenorrhea. Secondary amenorrhea is the most common finding in postpubertal women with hypogonadism and is the result of a reversible functional hypothalamic dysfunction.[4,5] Functional hypothalamic amenorrhea is a common cause of infertility, commonly triggered by excessive exercise, nutritional deficiencies, and psychological stressors.[5] Typical clinical manifestations of functional hypothalamic amenorrhea include amenorrhea for 6 months or longer, low to normal gonadotropin levels, and low serum estrogen levels.[5]

Primary ovarian failure is often caused by developmental defects such as ovarian agenesis, chromosomal abnormalities, and ovarian steroid production defects.[21] Other causes of primary hypogonadism include radiation, chemotherapy, and autoimmune diseases, which lead to premature ovarian failure.[21] The most common genetic cause of primary hypogonadism in women is Turner syndrome.[6] Turner syndrome is a chromosomal disorder that results when one set of genes from the short arm of the X chromosome is absent.[22] This chromosomal abnormality affects female development.[22] Short stature is the most common feature of Turner syndrome, and premature ovarian failure is also very common.[23] Initially, the ovaries develop normally, but premature death of the oocytes usually occurs and most of the ovarian tissue degenerates before birth.[23] Most women with Turner syndrome are infertile and many do not undergo puberty without hormone replacement therapy.[23] However, a small percentage of women with Turner syndrome maintain normal ovarian function through young adulthood.[23]

As with men, secondary hypogonadism in women is caused by a dysfunction in the hypothalamic–pituitary–gonadal axis.[1–5] Common causes of hypogonadotropic hypogonadism include anorexia nervosa, medications (ie, glucocorticoids and opiates), cessation of anabolic steroids, nutritional deficiencies, radiation, rapid, significant weight loss (including after bariatric surgery), trauma, and tumors.[4]

Diagnosis

Diagnosis of female hypogonadism is affected by onset, comorbidities, and severity of the dysfunction.[4,5] It is most often diagnosed in the first or second decade of life, during which time pubertal onset is expected.[5] Female patients with hypogonadism usually present with primary amenorrhea, underdeveloped breasts, short stature, eunuchoidism, or infertility.[4,5] Postpubertal clinical manifestations include secondary amenorrhea, hot flashes, decreased libido, changes in mood and energy levels, and osteoporosis.[4,5]

In addition to clinical presentation, diagnostic testing should be done, including estrogen level, FSH, LH, and pituitary function studies (**Fig. 2**).[4] Increased LH and FSH levels are consistent with primary ovarian failure.[24,25] Secondary ovarian failure is consistent with low LH and FSH levels and indicates a hypothalamic or pituitary dysfunction.[24,25] Additional, symptom driven laboratories may also be warranted. These tests include serum iron and prolactin levels, thyroid function studies, and karyotyping to assess for the presence of chromosomal abnormalities.[4] Antiovarian antibody levels should be checked in women with normal karyotype and elevated gonadotropin levels, to exclude autoimmune disease.[4] Total and free testosterone levels and 17-hydroxyprogesterone concentrations should be checked in postpubertal women presenting with acne, hirsutism, and/or amenorrhea or irregular menses.[4] Imaging studies may also be indicated in women with symptoms of hypogonadism. MRI of the hypothalamic-pituitary area should be done for suspected hypogonadotropic hypogonadism and to rule out or confirm pituitary involvement.[4,5] Pelvic ultrasound and/or MRI may be indicated to assess for ovarian abnormalities.[4] In

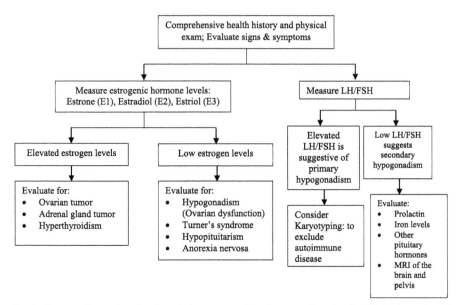

Fig. 2. Diagnostic workup for female hypogonadism. A comprehensive health history should be obtained at the initial visit to determine existence of systemic disorders, substance use/abuse (opioids, glucocorticoids, anabolic steroids), and eating disorders (ie, anorexia nervosa). Estrogenic hormone levels vary in women based on reproductive cycle and age. Reference ranges vary by laboratory; therefore, providers should use the ranges provided by the laboratory in their clinical practice. Prolactin levels guide diagnosis of prolactinoma. MRI should be ordered on a case-by-case basis and directly related to the patient's clinical presentation. (*Data from* Bhasin S, Cunningham GR, Hayes FJ, et al. Testosterone therapy in men with androgen deficiency syndromes: an endocrine society clinical practice guideline. J Clin Endocrinol Metab 2010;95(6):2536–59; and Hypogonadism. Medscape Web site. 2017. Available at: https://emedicine.medscape.com/article/922038. Accessed November 1, 2017.)

disorders of sexual development (DSD) cases, such as androgen insensitivity or ovotesticular DSD, an MRI of the pelvis is typically performed to aid in delineation of the anatomy of internal genitalia.[4]

Prognosis

As with men with hypogonadism, morbidity for women with hypogonadism includes negative effects on quality of life, infertility and its psychological effects, and osteoporosis.[4,26] Infertile women have higher levels of depression, anxiety, and stress than fertile women.[26] Many of the causes of hypogonadism are treatable and have positive outcomes.[4]

Screening

There is no evidence in the literature to support routine screening for hypogonadism.

Clinical Management

The goal of therapy for hypogonadal women is to induce and maintain secondary sex characteristics, normalize sexual function, and improve bone and muscle mass.[4,5,26] Therapy should be individualized for each patient, and is guided by age of onset, growth and growth potential, and the patient's psychosocial needs.[4] Young women with bone ages at or less than 12 years should be started on a very low starting dose of estrogen, because higher doses may cause rapid epiphyseal maturation.[4]

The standard treatment for women with hypogonadism is hormone replacement therapy with estrogen (**Table 2**).[4,5,26] Available estrogen replacement options include oral and transdermal. Natural estrogens, as opposed to synthetic, are the treatment of choice due to incomplete metabolism of synthetic estrogens, which increases the risk for thromboembolism and arterial hypertension.[5] Several estrogen-progesterone combination oral contraceptives can be used as replacement therapy for female patients with hypogonadism. Patient education should include all contraindications, precautions, and drug interactions for estrogens and progesterones.[4,5]

Oral or transdermal estradiol is the recommended treatment for induction of puberty in young women (see **Table 2**).[4,5] The recommended initial oral estrogen therapy is with a small, unopposed daily dose for 3 to 6 months, after which time the dose is increased and cycled.[4] The initial transdermal dose may be titrated after 6 to 12 months.[4] Adding progestogen after the first 6 months is recommended to aid in cyclical therapy (see **Table 2**).[4,5]

Although hormone replacement is the primary treatment for hypogonadism, individual patient needs and management of other effects of the disorder must be considered. Women with hypogonadotropic hypogonadism are at increased risk for poor skeletal development, bone loss, and fracture. Therefore, in addition to hormone replacement, clinical management should include calcium and vitamin D

Table 2
Hypogonadism management in women

	Route	Dosing	Therapeutic Effect	Patient Education
Prepubertal estrogen therapy options: • Ethinyl estradiol or • Conjugated equine estrogen or • Micronized estradiol	Oral Oral Oral	• 5 µg daily • 0.15–0.3 mg daily • 0.5 mg daily Titrate estrogen dose upward in 6–12 mo intervals to 0.625 mg, over a 2–3 y period.[4,5,21]	Promotes breast development and induction of puberty	Advise patient to report the following immediately: • Abdominal pain • Chest pain and shortness of breath • Sudden/ persistent headaches
Full hormone replacement therapy: • Conjugated equine estrogen Combined with: • Medroxyprogesterone acetate or • Micronized progesterone	Oral Oral Oral	• 0.625–1.25 mg daily • 5–10 mg daily • 200 mg	Menses induction; Cyclical therapy (Initiate after 6 mo or when breakthrough bleeding occurs)[4,5]	• Eye problems • Severe leg pain and/or swelling of the ankles and feet
Other treatment options: • Micronized estradiol • 17β-Estradiol patches • Estrogen gel	Oral Transdermal Transdermal	• 2 mg daily • 100–200 µg 1–2 times/wk • 1–2 mg daily	Induction of puberty	

Data from Refs.[4,5,26]

supplements, along with nutritional counseling.[5] Low-dose testosterone or the male hormone dehydroepiandrosterone may be prescribed for women with hypogonadism who experience decreased libido.[4]

Controversies

Long-term use of hormone therapy can increase the risk of breast cancer, blood clots, and heart disease.[4] Therefore, patients who choose to receive hormone replacement therapy should be well informed by their health care provider regarding the risks and benefits of hormone replacement therapy. Implications for future research and publication exist due to limited published literature on female hypogonadism.

SUMMARY

Current research supports the notion that testosterone replacement therapy is more beneficial than harmful, and this should be considered in the management of hypogonadism in men. Because of the complicated nature of hypogonadism, interprofessional collaboration is of great benefit to these patients. The psychosocial impact of hypogonadism in men and women must become a clinical management priority.

REFERENCES

1. Bhasin S, Cunningham GR, Hayes FJ, et al. Testosterone therapy in men with androgen deficiency syndromes: an Endocrine Society clinical practice guideline. J Clin Endocrinol Metab 2010;95(6):2536–59.
2. Bhasin S, Basaria B. Diagnosis and treatment of hypogonadism in men. Best Pract Res Clin Endocrinol Metab 2011;25(2):251–70.
3. Basaria S. Male hypogonadism. Lancet 2014;383:1250–63.
4. Hypogonadism. Medscape Web site. 2017. Available at: https://emedicine.medscape.com/article/922038. Accessed November 1, 2017.
5. Silveira LFG, Latronico C. Approach to the patient with hypogonadotropic hypogonadism. J Clin Endocrinol Metab 2013;98(5):1781–8.
6. Stamou MI, Georgopoulos NA. Kallman syndrome: phenotype and genotype of hypogonadotropic hypogonadism. Metabolism 2017. https://doi.org/10.1016/j.metabol.2017.10.012.
7. Gianetta E, Gianfrilli D, Barbagallo F, et al. Subclinical male hypogonadism. Best Pract Res Clin Endocrinol Metab 2012;26:539–50.
8. Traish AM. Benefits and health implications of testosterone therapy in men with testosterone deficiency. Sex Med Rev 2018;6(1):86–105.
9. Traish A, Haider A, Haider KS, et al. Long-term testosterone therapy improves cardiometabolic function and reduces risk of cardiovascular disease in men with hypogonadism: a real-life observational registry study setting comparing treated and untreated (control) groups. J Cardiovasc Pharmacol Ther 2017; 22(5):414–33.
10. Li H, Mitchell L, Zhang X, et al. Testosterone therapy and the risk of acute myocardial infarction in hypogonadal men: an administrative health care claims study. J Sex Med 2017;14:1307–17.
11. Loo SY, Chen BY, Yu OHY, et al. Testosterone replacement therapy and the risk of stroke in men: a systematic review. Maturitas 2017;106:31–7.
12. Morgentaler A, Miner MM, Caliber M, et al. Testosterone therapy and cardiovascular risks: advances and controversies. Mayo Clin Proc 2015;90(2):224–51.

13. Morgentaler A, Zitzmann M, Traish AM, et al. Fundamental concepts regarding testosterone deficiency and treatment: international expert consensus resolutions. Mayo Clin Proc 2016;91(7):881–96.
14. Goodman N, Guay A, Dandona P, et al, AACE Reproductive Endocrinology Scientific Committee. American Association of Clinical Endocrinologists and American College of Endocrinology position statement on the association of testosterone and cardiovascular risks. Endocr Pract 2015;21(9):1066–73.
15. Baillargeon J, Urban RJ, Kuo YF, et al. Risk of myocardial infarction in older men receiving testosterone therapy. Ann Pharmacother 2014;48(9):1138–44.
16. Baillargeon J, Urban RJ, Morgantaler A, et al. Risk of venous thromboembolism in men receiving testosterone therapy. Mayo Clin Proc 2015;90(8):1038–45.
17. Sharma R, Oni OA, Gupta K, et al. Normalization of testosterone level is associated with reduced incidence of myocardial infarction and mortality in men. Eur Heart J 2015;36(40):2706–15.
18. Tan RS, Cook KR, Reilly WG. Myocardial infarction and stroke risk in young healthy men treated with injectable testosterone. Int J Endocrinol 2015;2015:970750.
19. Etminan M, Skeldon SC, Goldenberg SL, et al. Testosterone therapy and risk of myocardial infarction: a pharmacoepidemiologic study. Pharmacotherapy 2015;35(1):72–8.
20. Anderson JL, May HT, Lappé DL, et al. Impact of testosterone replacement therapy on myocardial infarction, stroke, and death in men with low testosterone concentrations in an integrated health care system. Am J Cardiol 2016;117(5):794–9.
21. Estrogens. Lab tests online Web site. 2001-2017. Available at: https://labtestsonline.org/tests/estrogens. Accessed November 15, 2017.
22. Daniel MS, Postellon DC. 2017 Turner Syndrome. Medscape Web site. Available at: https://emedicine.medscape.com/article/949681-overview. Accessed February 14, 2018.
23. Turner Syndrome. National Institutes of Health U.S. National Library of Medicine Genetics Home reference Web site. 2017. Available at: https://ghr.nlm.nih.gov/condition/turner-syndrome. Accessed October 3, 2017.
24. Luteinizing hormone. Lab tests online Web site. 2001-2017. Available at: https://labtestsonline.org/tests/estrogens. Accessed November 15, 2017.
25. Follicle stimulating hormone. Lab tests online Web site. 2001-2017. Available at: https://labtestsonline.org/tests/estrogens. Accessed November 15, 2017.
26. Dzemaili S, Tiemensma J, Quinton R, et al. Beyond hormone replacement: quality of life in women with congenital hypogonadotropic hypogonadism. Endocr Connect 2016;6:404–12.

Polycystic Ovary Syndrome

Renate K. Meier, MS, MSN, WHNP-BC, SANE-A

KEYWORDS

- Polycystic ovary syndrome • Subtypes/phenotypes • Diagnosis • Management
- Treatment • Women's health • Hyperandrogenism • Anovulation

KEY POINTS

- Polycystic ovary syndrome (PCOS) is the most commonly occurring endocrine disorder among women with wide-reaching consequences that affect every aspect of a woman's life, including her reproductive, mental, cardiovascular, and metabolic health.
- Current understanding of PCOS outside of obstetrics and gynecology is limited, and it is often these providers who are tasked with the management of the vast metabolic and cardiovascular sequelae of the syndrome.
- There are several diagnostic criteria for PCOS, but all conclude that hyperandrogenism and ovulatory dysfunction are key components of the disorder.
- Treatment is focused on symptom relief and should be patient centered and undertaken in a multidisciplinary fashion to minimize the long-term risks of the syndrome.

BACKGROUND AND INTRODUCTION

Polycystic ovary syndrome (PCOS) is the most common endocrine disorder among women with a world-wide incidence estimated to be in the range of 4% to 12%.[1,2] Since the establishment of a more standardized diagnostic criteria in 1990, and with the ongoing revision of said criteria, the incidence of PCOS has been increasing in the United States and is now predicted to be closer to 18%.[3,4] Although there are several criteria from various specialty societies present for evaluation and characterization of PCOS, they are all in agreement that certain factors be present, including biochemical or clinical hyperandrogenism and ovulatory dysfunction, such as chronic oligo-ovulation or anovulation.[3] Polycystic ovaries have also been associated with the syndrome but are no longer required for diagnosis, and similarly the presence of insulin resistance and hyperinsulinemia is common among women with PCOS but are again not required for diagnosis.[5] Further, because PCOS is a syndrome encompassing a constellation of symptoms, there is no single diagnostic test available for the diagnosis of the disorder and there is neither a single consequence nor organ system

Disclosure Statement: The author has nothing to disclose.
Department of Obstetrics and Gynecology, Vanderbilt University School of Medicine, Vanderbilt University Medical Center, 1161 21st Avenue South, Nashville, TN 37232, USA
E-mail address: rkmeier01@gmail.com

Nurs Clin N Am 53 (2018) 407–420
https://doi.org/10.1016/j.cnur.2018.04.008
0029-6465/18/© 2018 Elsevier Inc. All rights reserved.

affected by the disorder. Although traditionally viewed through the lens of a reproductive disorder, evidence emerging since the late 1990s has supported that PCOS places women at an increased risk for the development of cardiovascular and metabolic disorders, thus, making PCOS a significant contributor to women's health issues across multiple specialties and in all stages of life[6] and leading some to suggest the disorder be renamed to "metabolic reproductive syndrome" (Sheila E. Laredo, MD, PhD, University of Toronto).[7]

The fact that PCOS is recognized mainly within the obstetrics and gynecology specialty and is poorly understood by those in other specialties and in primary care has led to major barriers to effective and comprehensive health care for women, as they are often racing from one provider to the next for their care. In one population-based study, it was demonstrated that 68% of women meeting the diagnostic criteria for PCOS remained undiagnosed[8]; these are women who are at high risk for the development of diabetes, cardiovascular disease, and metabolic disorders, which are managed outside of the obstetrics and gynecology specialty. Women who rely on internists and family practitioners for long-term risk reduction interventions and yet the practitioners they rely on are likely unfamiliar with their syndrome and how to screen for and manage it appropriately.[7] The most effective management of the complex reproductive, cardiovascular, and metabolic sequelae these women face will come from collaboration of providers across a wide range of specialties who will each contribute their expertise, but for now we can aim to increase education among various specialties of the diagnostic criteria for PCOS and basic management strategies so that all providers are at least minimally comfortable in generating a diagnosis and beginning the treatment process.

DEFINING POLYCYSTIC OVARY SYNDROME

Historically, PCOS has been characterized by a constellation of symptoms and clinical features, including hyperandrogenism (acne, hirsutism, hyperinsulinemia), menstrual irregularities (cycle length >35 days, oligo-ovulation or anovulation), and/or polycystic ovaries. Keeping in line with these general clinical features, there have been several proposed diagnostic criteria for PCOS as described in **Table 1**.[3,9,10]

Although the use of such classification systems has been beneficial to some degree for strengthening our understanding of the syndrome, it has, at the same time, created

Table 1
Proposed diagnostic criteria for polycystic ovarian syndrome

Criteria	NIH 1990	Rotterdam	AE-PCOS

Hyperandrogenism
  Clinical: acne, hirsutism, alopecia
    (Ferriman-Gallwey score >8)
  Biochemical: elevated total/free testosterone
	+	+/−	+

Oligo-ovulation/anovulation
  ≤6–9 menstrual cycles per year
  Cycle length >35 d
  Day 21 progesterone documenting anovulation
	+	+/−	+/−

Polycystic ovaries
  12+ antral follicles 2–9 mm in a single ovary
  Total ovarian volume >10 mL
	...	+/−	+/−

Abbreviations: AE-PCOS, Androgen Excess and Polycystic Ovary Syndrome Society; NIH, National Institutes of Health.

a more convoluted system that has hindered the ability of clinicians to appropriately partner with women to address their individual health issues and concerns and has also delayed our progress on the syndrome.[11] Specifically, with the broadening of the diagnostic criteria for PCOS brought about by the Rotterdam and Androgen Excess and Polycystic Ovary Syndrome Society criteria, multiple phenotypes of women with PCOS were included into studies without stratification based on phenotype.[7] This inclusion created significant confusion because features of the syndrome vary by phenotype, most notably the metabolic features.[7] For that reason, it has been recommended that specific subtypes be addressed in literature. Furthermore, it has been proposed that treatments should be directed toward phenotype as well. Based on the Rotterdam criteria, the most widely used and most relevant criteria for diagnosis, there are 4 phenotypes/subtypes of PCOS that can be identified shown in **Table 2**: (1) frank/classic PCOS (hyperandrogenism, oligo-ovulation/anovulation with polycystic-appearing ovaries or H-O-P), (2) non-polycystic ovary PCOS (hyperandrogenism, oligo-ovulation/anovulation with normal-appearing ovaries or H-A), (3) ovulatory PCOS (hyperandrogenism and polycystic-appearing ovaries with regular menstrual cycles or H-P), and (4) mild or normo-androgenic PCOS (oligo-ovulation/anovulation with polycystic-appearing ovaries and normal androgen levels) with prevalences of 66%, 11%, 13%, and 9%.[12,13] Furthermore, evidence supports that women with subtypes 2 and 4 have a lower incidence of chronic diseases (decreased incidence of abdominal obesity, insulin resistance, and inflammation); those with ovulatory PCOS have lower risks of endometrial cancer, whereas those with frank PCOS have the most severe metabolic disturbances.[13] It is important to note, however, that metabolic disturbances continued to depend on body mass index (BMI); thus, dietary and lifestyle modifications and interventions among this population in particular are crucial for syndrome management.[13]

CLINICAL FEATURES AND DIAGNOSTIC CRITERIA

Health care concerns for women with PCOS tend to be focused on reproductive function as well as on management of hirsutism, alopecia, and acne.[14] The actual clinical presentation will vary depending on the subtype as well as age and lifestyle factors of the patients. Women can be completely without symptoms or may present with any of several complaints, including dermatologic issues such as hirsutism and acne, irregular menses, and infertility.[5]

More than 80% of women presenting with signs and symptoms of androgen excess have PCOS.[5,15] In adult women, clinical signs of hyperandrogenism can

Table 2
Rotterdam phenotypes of polycystic ovarian syndrome

Criteria	Classic	2	3	4

Hyperandrogenism
   Clinical: acne, hirsutism, alopecia (Ferriman-Gallwey score >8)
   Biochemical: elevated total/free testosterone
	+	+	+	…

Oligo-ovulation/anovulation
   ≤6–9 menstrual cycles per year
   Cycle length >35 d
   Day 21 progesterone documenting anovulation
	+	+	…	+

Polycystic ovaries
   12+ antral follicles 2–9 mm in a single ovary
   Total ovarian volume >10 mL
	+	…	+	+

be measured through physical examination and are typically acceptable for diagnosis of PCOS. These signs would include hirsutism, alopecia and acne and should be considered as indicating a condition of excess androgen production.[14] Hirsutism is a condition defined by the increased presence of terminal hairs versus vellus hairs and in PCOS is typically more pronounced over the chin, neck, lower face, and sideburns (especially if medially extending). Further, excessive hair growth is often observed across the lower back, abdomen, buttocks, perineal area, inner thighs, and peri-areolar areas as well. Hirsutism tends to develop gradually and intensifies with weight gain.[14] Most commonly, modified Ferriman-Gallwey scoring is used to assess hirsutism. (Hair growth is evaluated across several sites and scored 0 for absence of terminal hair to 4 for excessive presence of terminal hair; scores >8 indicate hirsutism.)[5] In addition to presenting with hirsutism, women with PCOS often exhibit alopecia. Typically, PCOS-associated alopecia presents as male pattern hair loss developing at the vertex, crown, or in a diffuse pattern; but those with severe hyperandrogenemia may develop bitemporal and frontline hair loss.[14] Finally, when acne is present after adolescence or is exacerbated suddenly in the mid-20s or mid-30s, it can be a clinical sign of hyperandrogenism and elevated serum testosterone.[14,16] Although, acne is less prevalent in PCOS and less specific an indicator than hirsutism, as only 15% to 30% of adult women with PCOS present with acne.[5]

Ovulatory dysfunction and menstrual irregularities are common among women with PCOS. A cycle length greater than 35 days suggests anovulation and is associated with an increased risk for development of endometrial hyperplasia and cancer[17] as well as infertility.[14] In women with oligomenorrhea, 85% to 90% will have PCOS, whereas 30% to 40% of women with amenorrhea will have PCOS.[5] Further, in women with amenorrhea presenting to fertility clinics for care, 90% to 95% have PCOS.[5] In these women, the mechanism of infertility is related to the arrest of follicular development, so they tend to have a normal number of primordial follicles with increased numbers of primary and secondary follicles and a lack of development of a dominant follicle.[18] In addition to having more difficulty in becoming pregnant, women with PCOS have been demonstrated to have a more difficult time in sustaining pregnancies, with a first-trimester miscarriage rate at 30% to 50%.[19]

As previously mentioned, the presence of insulin resistance and hyperinsulinemia is common among women with PCOS; although not required to make the diagnosis of PCOS, hyperinsulinemic insulin resistance has been demonstrated to play a prominent role in PCOS,[5] with up to 80% of women with PCOS demonstrating insulin resistance in one large clinical study.[20] Further, the prevalence of insulin resistance in PCOS occurs independently of obesity, although the effect of obesity on insulin resistance is additive to that of PCOS.[5,20] Although most women with PCOS are able to maintain beta cell function, as many as 30% to 40% will go on to develop impaired glucose tolerance and 7.5% to 10.0% type 2 diabetes.[5]

There are many additional health concerns among women with PCOS. Metabolic syndrome is also more common in women with PCOS, with the prevalence being twice that compared with the general population.[21] Nonalcoholic fatty liver disease,[21] sleep apnea,[21] hypertension,[5] and dyslipidemia[5,21] are also more prevalent in women with PCOS, even when the BMI is controlled for. Cerebrovascular disease and cardiovascular disease but not cardiovascular mortality are increased consistently in studies of women with PCOS.[21] Finally, there have been some studies that correlate mental health disorders with PCOS, demonstrating a higher frequency of depression, drug disorders, bipolar disorder, bulimia, anorexia, and other nonspecific eating disorders[6] in women with PCOS.[4]

DIAGNOSTIC WORKUP

For patients presenting with signs or symptoms of PCOS, the diagnostic workup should always begin with a thorough history and physical examination (HPE) with a focus on menstrual history, signs of hirsutism (acne, alopecia, acanthosis nigricans, skin tags), and weight and its interplay on the aforementioned symptoms.[21] Because the diagnosis of PCOS by the Rotterdam criteria requires 2 of 3 findings (hyperandrogenism, ovulatory dysfunction, or polycystic ovaries), diagnosis can typically be accomplished with HPE and basic laboratory testing without the need for ultrasonography or other imaging.[21] However, for the most effective risk stratification and to identify the PCOS subtype, ultrasonography would be required.

In terms of menstrual history, for women presenting with oligomenorrhea (cycle length >35 days but <6 months[22]) may be assumed to have chronic anovulation.[14] If, however, cycles are slightly longer (32–35 days) or are irregular (varying from 32–36 days), ovulation should be assessed. Further, in hyperandrogenic women with normal-appearing cycles, there is a chance that cycles are anovulatory as well, so it is recommended that ovulation be assessed in these women as well.[14] The gold standard for determination of ovulation is to measure midluteal phase progesterone when levels greater than 10 ng/mL indicate regular luteal function.[14] Alternatively, basal body temperature charts, urinary luteinizing hormone (LH) kits, or timed endometrial biopsies may be used; but their usefulness is limited, as the information they produce is incomplete.[14]

There has been some controversy in the literature regarding which hormones should be included in the workup for PCOS, typically varying depending on which specialty is consulted and also differing in regard to which biochemical assays are accepted as useful in defining hyperandrogenism. Classically, practitioners were advised to check thyroid-stimulating hormone (TSH), prolactin (PRL), follicle-stimulating hormone (FSH), LH, dehydroepiandrosterone (DHEA), DHEA sulfate (DHEAS), and total and free testosterone (T) with advice that a ratio of LH:FSH near 2:1 with elevated levels of androgenic hormones correlated to a diagnosis of PCOS, which is what many primary care specialties continue to teach.[21] The American College of Obstetrics and Gynecology currently recommends screening for biochemical hyperandrogenism with either total T and sex hormone–binding globulin (SHBG) or bioavailable and free T with exclusion of other causes of hyperandrogenism via TSH, PRL, and 17-hydroxyprogesterone (17-OHP), and screening for metabolic abnormalities with a 2-hour oral glucose tolerance test as well as fasting lipid and lipoprotein levels.[23] However, current specialty recommendations are to evaluate only free T, 17-OHP, and anti-müllerian hormone (AMH).[9,14]

Chemically, hyperandrogenism is characterized by elevated levels to total, bioavailable, or free T or DHEAS. However, in patients with PCOS, the value of measuring androgens other than T is low, especially when considering the cost of these assays. Although DHEAS may be elevated in 30% to 35% of women with PCOS, measurement of DHEAS adds nothing to the diagnosis, as in most patients free and total T are also increased.[14] The use of further androgen testing would be for exclusion of other treatable conditions that mimic PCOS, such as to eliminate androgen-secreting tumors in patients with rapid-onset symptoms.[21] Thus, the recommendation is to measure free T either directly by equilibrium dialysis or through a calculation based on the total T measured accurately by radioimmunoassay using a purified sample.[14,23]

In women with PCOS, measurement of prolactin levels often reveals mild-moderate elevations[23] and is recommended to rule out prolactinomas, an extremely rare cause of hyperandrogenic chronic anovulation. Similarly, evaluation of TSH levels is recommended, as thyroid disease is frequently associated with menstrual disorders and ovarian dysregulation.[23] Further fasting 17-OHP is beneficial as a screening tool for nonclassic congenital adrenal hyperplasia.[23] Women with 21-hydroxylase deficiency can present with hyperandrogenism and anovulation; a normal value is less than 2 ng/mL, and greater than 10 ng/mL indicates a deficiency.[14]

Transvaginal ultrasonography should be used for the evaluation of ovarian morphology.[14] The existing Rotterdam criteria have defined polycystic ovary morphology as the presence of at least 12 follicles between 2 and 9 mm in a single ovary or by measurement of increased ovarian volume with size greater than 10 mL.[24] However, new technology has since become available; when using this technology (software for automatic follicle numbering in conjunction with probes with an 8 mHz or greater frequency), the threshold for ovarian follicle count has been increased to 25.[14] In instances in which the clinician is not aware about the technology used, only ovarian size rather than follicle count should be used for diagnosis. Eventually, AMH values may be added to corroborate ovarian volume.[14]

OUTLINE OF MANAGEMENT STRATEGIES FOR POLYCYSTIC OVARY SYNDROME

The treatment modality applied to a particular patient with PCOS depends primarily on her goals and the desired clinical effect of treatment: alleviation of the symptoms of hyperandrogenism, regulation of menstrual dysfunction, or treatment of infertility.[5,6,21] Further, optimal results will require a patient-centered multidisciplinary approach involving primary care and subspecialty providers who partner with a woman to help her achieve her treatment goals.[21]

Treatment of Androgen-Related Symptoms

As previously discussed, the most commonly associated complaints of hyperandrogenism among women with PCOS are hirsutism, acne, and alopecia; typically oral contraceptives (OCPs) are the first-line treatment in premenopausal patients.[5] Because of the growth cycle of the hair follicle, patients should be counseled that it can take 6 months or more to produce pharmacologic results and after that period if no improvement is noted antiandrogens can be added.[5] In terms of which OCP works best, evidence has demonstrated that pills with daily doses of ethinyl estradiol (EE) of 20 to 35 mcg (or combined OCP [COCs]) function 3-fold to suppress the decreased androgen production: first, they increase SHBG levels, which results in suppression of ovarian androgen production[5,14]; second, they reduce adrenal androgen production[5,14]; and third, they prevent peripheral conversion of T into the more potent dihydrotestosterone (DHT) as well as act as competitive inhibitors of DHT at the androgen receptors.[5,14] Further, there has been a refinement of progestins to create more desirable profiles with greater progestogenic and less androgenic activities. In women with PCOS, the ideal progestin is that with the lowest androgenic profile, such as drospirenone.[5] Thus, for women with PCOS without contraindications to COCs, EE/drospirenone-type pills, such as Yaz or Yasmin, would have the best profile according to these standards.

Spironolactone and flutamide have also been limitedly demonstrated to be effective for the management of hirsutism associated with PCOS.[14,21] Spironolactone functions primarily through antagonism of the androgen receptor, but it also inhibits ovarian and adrenal steroidogenesis, directly inhibits 5-alpha-reductase activity, and antagonizes androgen receptors within hair follicles.[5,14] Typically, spironolactone is used at a dosage of 100 mg daily but may be titrated up to 200 mg daily in divided doses, whereas flutamide is given as 250 mg twice daily.[5,14,21] Less commonly, dexamethasone or prednisone can be used to directly lower androgen output.[14]

Other therapies for hirsutism include the application of Vaniqa cream, electrolysis, or light-based therapies, such as laser hair removal or pulse light therapy.[6,21] Although for androgenic alopecia, it is recommended that 5-alpha reductase inhibitors, such as finasteride, be given.[6]

And for acne, COCs alone or in conjunction with topical retinoids have demonstrated effectiveness in treatment with the addition of antiandrogens considered to be second-line therapy.[21]

Treatment of Menstrual-Related Disorders

For patients with PCOS presenting with menstrual irregularities not seeking fertility, OCPs should be the first-line therapy, as they effectively restore cyclic bleeding, reduce hyperandrogenism, and reduce the risk of endometrial hyperplasia.[5,6,14,21,23] There have been some studies demonstrating metformin restores normal menstruation in 50% to 70% of women with PCOS[21]; however, OCPs have been shown superior for menstrual regulation as well as for lowering androgen levels. The goal with irregular bleeding is prevention of endometrial hyperplasia from chronic anovulation/unopposed estrogen stimulation of the endometrium. In a joint meeting of the European Society of Human Reproduction and Embryology and the American Society for Reproductive Medicine, it was recommended that menstrual flow be initiated at least every 3 months.[25] In addition to the use of OCPs, progesterone derivatives may be administered every 90 days to initiate a withdrawal bleed or patients may select levonorgestrel-releasing intrauterine systems.[21,23]

Fertility Challenges and Care

For women with PCOS, fertility tends to be a large hurdle in not only their health care but also in obtaining optimal quality of life. Women with PCOS tend to struggle with infertility and make up a large portion of patients within the fertility clinic setting.[5] Traditionally, weight loss and lifestyle modification have been the recommended first-line therapy for these women.[5,21] It was thought that because there was a correlation between anovulation and pregnancy loss and obesity that recommending weight loss would improve a woman's chances at conceiving and continuing a pregnancy, and so clinicians have been taught to teach women with body image and weight issues that their weight is the issue in this arena as well. There was even evidence that showed weight loss of 5% to 10% increased ovulation and bariatric surgery improved cycle regularity and increased ovulation.[26–28] Although weight loss has been shown to have a positive effect on fertility, current research fails to show any effect of lifestyle modification on pregnancy rates.[29]

Rather than preaching weight loss and a calorie-restricted diet at women who likely already have body image issues and depression related to infertility, it would better serve all parties involved for clinicians to follow evidence-based practices and prescribe either clomiphene citrate (CC; Clomid) or letrozole (Femara) for ovulation induction.[5,6,14,21,30] When measuring the only outcome that matters to patients, birth of a live infant, recent studies demonstrate letrozole to have higher live birth rates; thus, it is becoming preferred over CC.[31,32] Similarly to weight loss, the impact of metformin on fertility has become controversial since a Cochrane review published in 2012 concluded there is no evidence to support that metformin improves fertility as was once thought.[30,33]

With CC, ovulation induction occurs when CC binds to estrogen receptors to inhibit negative feedback signaling at the level of the hypothalamus thereby increasing gonadotropin secretion to trigger ovulation.[34–36] This method is, in fact, highly effective producing ovulation rates that range between 70% and 85% per cycle as measured in some studies[36,37]; however, the pregnancy rate with Clomid is only 20%, related to the antiestrogenic properties of Clomid at the level of the endometrium and the negative effects on cervical mucus.[36,37] Regimens are recommended to begin with 50-mg daily dosing on cycle days 2 to 7, increasing 50 mg per cycle to a maximum dosage of 150 mg/d if ovulation does not occur.[38] It is important to note that with CC, pregnancy is typically achieved rapidly and effectively, with 75% of pregnancies occurring in the first 3 months, so consider alternative treatment or referral if results are not seen.[6]

Letrozole, an aromatase inhibitor, has shown promise in use as an ovulation induction agent. Unlike Clomid, Femara induces ovulation by blocking the conversion of androgens into estrogen, lowering the estrogen levels to reduce negative feedback and increasing gonadotropin production.[35] Because Femara does not bind directly to the estrogen receptors, it lacks the antiestrogenic properties of Clomid and is suspected to be less detrimental to the endometrial lining and cervical mucus, which has in turn led to the proposal that pregnancy rates with Femara may surpass those achieved with Clomid.[35–37] In fact, recent studies have resulted in some researchers suggesting that Femara replace Clomid as the first-line therapy for ovulation induction in women with PCOS.[31,32,37] Regimens are recommended to begin with 5-mg daily dosing on cycle days 2 to 7, increasing 2.5 mg per cycle to a maximum dosage of 10.0 mg to 12.5 mg/d if ovulation does not occur.[30–32] Once again pregnancy should be achieved rapidly, and after 6 months patients should be referred on for alternative management.

SUMMARY

Women with PCOS make up a significant part of the population worldwide; because of a lack of complete understanding of the pathophysiology of the condition and because of its complexities management of this syndrome to date has been underwhelming. This circumstance is due in part to a lack of understanding of the complex pathophysiology of the condition, which you will notice is intentionally left uncovered in this review. Further complicating management to date has been the fact that because we do not fully understand the cause of PCOS, we cannot apply typical cause-and-effect-style treatments that are applied in other areas of practice to ideally address health. Instead, we are left treating individual symptoms of a disorder rather than the entire syndrome.

What we do know and understand is that there is no single diagnostic test for PCOS and there is no single presentation of the disorder. Further, we understand that women with the disorder have greater risks to their overall health, not just their reproductive health. They are at greater risk of metabolic and cardiovascular diseases and complications; thus, proper and early identification of these women is essential not only to their health but to the overall health of our population. Further, because health promotion of the population in general is central to the role of the nurse and nurse practitioner and in fact differentiates our profession from other medical professions, for example, doctors of medicine, physician assistants, and doctors of osteopathy,[39] management of these patients by a multidisciplinary team including nurse practitioners only makes sense, with improvement in lifestyle having the potential for a wide impact on both the quality and quantity of life in these women.[7] Thus, we are in a unique position to be able to promote a more comprehensive patient-centered model of care for this population. We can aim to increase education among various specialties of the diagnostic criteria for PCOS we can teach a comprehensive care approach with regular checkups and can promote teaching of lifestyle modifications in appropriate settings while eliminating it from areas where evidence has demonstrated it to be ineffective and we can together come up with best possible model to bridge to the day when the syndrome if fully understood and research has improved treatment success and overall patient management.

CASE STUDY 1: FRANK OR CLASSIC POLYCYSTIC OVARY SYNDROME

Subjective: A 23-year-old G0P0 white woman presents to an outpatient gynecologic (GYN) clinic with chief complaints of weight gain, excessive hair growth, and irregular menses. She has no known drug allergies (NKDA); currently uses no prescription, over-the-counter, or recreational drugs; and reports her last menstrual period (LMP) such that she is on cycled day 20 at presentation to the clinic.

History of present illness: The patient reports menarche at around at 13 years of age with regularity established at 17 years of age. She indicates her cycle length is between 35 and 40 days, lasting 3 days with very light bleeding (4 pads per day on a heavy day). She also reports a large weight gain and expresses difficulty with losing weight. She indicates attempts at weight regulation through diet and exercise, including structured programs like Weight Watchers and Jenny Craig, indicating that although she did experience weight loss, it was minimal and much less than was expected. She complains of facial hair, hair on her chest and abdomen, and mild acne over her face, chest, and back.

Past medical history: She reports childhood asthma but has not required an inhaler since 14 years of age and has had no major hospitalizations, no major illnesses, and no major injuries. Wisdom teeth extraction is her only surgical report; her immunizations are up to date, including human papillomavirus (HPV).

Family history: The only relevant family history is that her mother had difficulty trying to conceive but was unsure as to what the initial problem was. Her mother was eventually able to have children; once her first child was born, she did not have any further issues. She was able to have 4 children.

Review of systems: General: She reports a weight gain of 80 lb over 2 years; skin, hair, nails: She has acne that worsens with cycles and excessive hair growth on her face, chest, and abdomen; all other systems are negative (lymphatic, immune: no lumps or bumps, no excessive colds; HEENT: no vision problems, no headaches, no nasal drainage, no sore throats, no problems with hearing; cardiovascular [CV]: no palpitations, no chest pain, no previous cholesterol screening; respiratory: no shortness of breath, no cough; breast: monthly self-exams performed, no nipple discharge, no lumps/bumps/masses; gastrointestinal [GI]: no reflux, constipation, diarrhea; genitourinary [GU]: no burning, leaking, or urgency; neuromuscular [NM]: no muscle aches, no joint tenderness; endocrine: no feelings hot/cold, no fatigue, no previous screening tests; psychological: no anxiety, no depression, no drug abuse; neurologic: no numbness, no tingling, no headaches).

Objective

Physical examination findings: The patient is a 23-year-old G0P0 white woman with a height of 5 ft 2 in and weight of 233 lb, with a BMI of 42.6. She is well-groomed appearing and in no acute distress. She is very interactive/engaged during the examination with a pleasant mood, good eye contact, with speech of moderate pace. Her skin is warm, dry, and intact with moderate acne on the face and chest as well as some acanthosis nigracans at the back of the neck but no other discolorations noted. Her hair is moderately thin on the scalp and curly but soft with a positive hirsutism score of 12. Her head and neck are normal in appearance, atraumatic, normocephalic, and no dandruff; her neck is supple and the thyroid is barely palpable without nodules or masses. The heart has a regular rate and rhythm, with no murmurs, rubs, or gallops and normal S1 and S2. The lungs are clear to auscultation bilaterally in all fields. The breasts have a normal adult contour, Tanner stage V, no masses, dimpling, or retractions, and no spontaneous nipple discharge. The abdomen is soft, nontender, rounded, and doughy. The vulva is within normal limits; the hair has been removed, and there are no infestations or follicular inflammations. The vagina is clear without abnormal discharge and is pink with rugated walls. The cervix is pink and nulliparous without lesions abnormal discharge or tenderness and is freely mobile. Uterus is freely mobile, nontender, smooth, and without masses in a mid-to-posterior position and is normal in size. The adnexa are nontender bilaterally with ovaries enlarged and firm.

Assessment and plan: The assessment is classic PCOS. The patient does not desire immediate fertility but would like a definitive diagnosis. Transvaginal ultrasound (TVUS) and laboratory tests (PRL, LH, FSH, hemoglobin A1c [HgbA1c], TSH, DHEAS, free and total T, SHBG, 17-OHP [the patient does not have a primary care physician]) are ordered. Pharmacologic management is initiated: Yaz and eflornithine hydrochloride (Vaniqa) cream.

Results of Testing

Summary of ultrasound findings: The overall impression was polycystic appearance of ovaries with a small amount of free fluid surrounding the right ovary. The endometrial thickness was 9.0 mm. The left ovary had a total volume of 8.4 mL and 6 follicles 6 to 9 mm in size. The right ovary had a total volume of 11.5 mL and 8 follicles 7 to 15 mm in size. Automated software was not used for follicle counting, and the probe frequency was 5 mHz.

Laboratory Results

Hormone	Reference Range	Unit of Measurement	Value
PRL	2.74–26.72	ng/mL	10.49
LH	1.20–12.86	mIU/mL	8.83
FSH	1.79–5.12	mIU/mL	5.58
TSH	0.34–5.60	mIU/mL	1.01
DHEAS	80–560	mcg/dL	497
Total T	10–52	ng/dL	36
Free T	0.9–9.1	pg/mL	9.3
SHBG	12.2–135.5	nmol/L	15.7
17-OHP	22–469	ng/dL	283
A1c	4.6–6.2	%	4.7

CASE STUDY 2: MILD OR NORMO-ANDROGENIC POLYCYSTIC OVARY SYNDROME

Subjective: A 29-year-old G0P0 white woman presents to an outpatient GYN clinic with a chief complaint of infertility for 9 months in the setting of highly irregular menses. She has NKDA; currently uses no prescription, over-the-counter, or recreational drugs; and reports her LMP such that she is on cycled day 40 at the initial presentation to the clinic.

History of present illness: The patient reports that at 16 years of age she still had not experienced menarche and so at that point she was placed on OCPs and began having regular cycles. She indicates she continued the use of OCPs until her 20s at which time she took a 6-month break and again had no menses. At that time, she was instructed to have a withdrawal bleed and was placed back onto OCPs, which she continued until recently. She reports that after marriage, she and her partner discussed expanding their family and came to the conclusion that she would cease use of COCs and that they would attempt pregnancy. She reports irregular cycles with lengths varying from 32 to 40 days but averaging greater than 35 days since cessation of OCPs and indicates when menses do occur they are typically very light. She reports regular unprotected intercourse with her spouse 3 or more times most weeks and has not achieved pregnancy.

Past medical history: She reports no major hospitalizations, no major illnesses, and no major injuries. Immunizations are up to date, including HPV; however, she is repeating the hepatitis B series because of insufficient titer levels following administration of the initial vaccine series.

Family history: Her maternal grandmother had a similar menstrual history but was able to conceive. Her paternal aunt had unexplained infertility. There is no other relevant family history.

Review of systems: The review of systems is negative except irregular menstrual cycles with premenstrual mood lability. General: The results are within normal limits and stable; skin, hair, nails: she denies excessive oiliness, acne, or hirsutism; all other systems are negative (lymphatic, immune: no lumps or bumps, no excessive colds; HEENT: no vision problems, no headaches, no nasal drainage, no sore throats, no problems with hearing; CV: no palpitations, no chest pain; no previous cholesterol screening; respiratory: no shortness of breath, no cough; breast: monthly self-exams performed, no nipple discharge, no lumps/bumps/masses; GI: no reflux, constipation, diarrhea; GU: no burning, leaking, or urgency; NM: no muscle aches, no joint tenderness; endocrine: no feelings hot/cold, no fatigue, no previous screening tests; psychological: no anxiety, no depression, no drug abuse; neurologic: no numbness, no tingling, no headaches).

Objective

Physical examination findings: The patient is a 29-year-old G0P0 white woman with a height of 5 ft 11 in and weight of 180 lb, with a BMI of 25.1. She is well-groomed appearing and in no acute distress. She has a pleasant mood, good eye contact, and speech of moderate pace. Her skin is warm, dry, and intact without acne, acanthosis nigricans, or other discolorations noted. Her hair is thick and full on the scalp, and there is not an inappropriate presence of terminal hairs across the body (modified Ferriman-Gallwey score is 0). Her head and neck are normal in appearance, atraumatic, normocephalic, with no dandruff; the neck is supple and the thyroid palpable without nodules or masses. The heart has a regular rate and rhythm, no murmurs, rubs, or gallops, and a normal S1 and S2. The lungs are clear to auscultation bilaterally in all fields. The breasts have a normal adult contour, Tanner stage V, with no masses, dimpling, or retractions and no spontaneous nipple discharge. The abdomen is soft and nontender. The vulva is within normal limits; the hair has been removed, and there are no infestations or follicular inflammations. The vagina is clear without abnormal discharge and is pink with rugated walls. The cervix is pink and nulliparous without lesions, abnormal discharge, or tenderness and is freely mobile. The uterus is freely mobile, nontender, smooth, and without masses in an anterior position and is normal in size. The adnexa are nontender bilaterally with ovaries enlarged and firm.

Assessment and plan: The history is consistent with chronic anovulation, and physical exam is not suspicious of hyperandrogenism. Immediate fertility is desired as is a definitive diagnosis. TVUS and laboratory tests (LH, FSH, HgbA1C, TSH, DHEAS, free

T, SHBG, and lipid panel) are ordered. Pharmacologic management is initiated: A withdrawal bleed was initiated with medroxyprogesterone acetate (Provera) 10 mg daily for 10 days, and laboratory tests were collected on cycle day 3. Two cycles were attempted without ovulation induction without a successful pregnancy, and then ovulation induction was initiated. Femara was used at 5 mg daily for cycle days 2 to 7 for 2 cycles without success, and then the patient was provided a referral to reproductive endocrinology and infertility for further intervention.

Results of Testing

Summary of ultrasound findings: The overall impression was polycystic appearance of ovaries with an average ovarian volume of 12 mL and a string-of-pearls appearance to the ovaries. Automated software was not used for follicle counting, and the probe frequency was 5 mHz.

Laboratory Results

Hormone	Reference Range	Unit of Measurement	Value
LH	2.4–12.6	mIU/mL	7.5
FSH	3.5–12.5	mIU/mL	6.1
TSH	0.450–4.5	mIU/mL	3.060
DHEAS	84.8–378.0	mcg/dL	159.7
Free direct T	0.0–4.2	pg/mL	0.5
SHBG	24.6–122.0	nmol/L	45.9
A1C	4.8–5.6	%	5.5
Cholesterol	100–199	mg/dL	157
HDL	>39	mg/dL	60
LDL	0–99	mg/dL	85
Triglycerides	0–149	mg/dL	61
VLDL	5–40	mg/dL	12

Abbreviations: HDL, high-density lipoprotein; LDL, low-density lipoprotein; VLDL, very low-density lipoprotein.

REFERENCES

1. Franik S, Kremer JA, Nelen WL, et al. Aromatase inhibitors for subfertile women with polycystic ovary syndrome. Cochrane Database Syst Rev 2014;(2):CD010287.
2. Sheehan MT. Polycystic ovarian syndrome: diagnosis and management. Clin Med Res 2004;2(1):13–27.
3. Rotterdam ESHRE/ASRM-Sponsored PCOS Consensus Workshop Group. Revised 2003 consensus on diagnostic criteria and long-term health risks related to polycystic ovary syndrome. Fertil Steril 2004;81(1):19–25.
4. Teede H, Deeks A, Moran L. Polycystic ovary syndrome: a complex condition with psychological, reproductive and metabolic manifestations that impacts on health across the lifespan. BMC Med 2010;8:41.
5. Sirmans SM, Pate KA. Epidemiology, diagnosis, and management of polycystic ovary syndrome. Clin Epidemiol 2013;6:1–13.
6. Yau TT, Ng NY, Cheung LP, et al. Polycystic ovary syndrome: a common reproductive syndrome with long-term metabolic consequences. Hong Kong Med J 2017;23(6):622–34.

7. Dunaif A, Fauser BC. Renaming PCOS–a two-state solution. J Clin Endocrinol Metab 2013;98(11):4325–8.
8. March WA, Moore VM, Willson KJ, et al. The prevalence of polycystic ovary syndrome in a community sample assessed under contrasting diagnostic criteria. Hum Reprod 2010;25(2):544–51.
9. Azziz R, Carmina E, Dewailly D, et al. The androgen excess and PCOS society criteria for the polycystic ovary syndrome: the complete task force report. Fertil Steril 2009;91(2):456–88.
10. Zawadzki JK, Dunaif A. Diagnostic criteria for polycystic ovary syndrome: towards a rational approach. Boston: Blackwell Scientific Publications; 1992. p. 377–84.
11. National Institutes of Health. Evidence-based methodology workshop on polycystic ovary syndrome executive summary. 2012.
12. Guastella E, Longo RA, Carmina E. Clinical and endocrine characteristics of the main polycystic ovary syndrome phenotypes. Fertil Steril 2010;94(6):2197–201.
13. Clark NM, Podolski AJ, Brooks ED, et al. Prevalence of polycystic ovary syndrome phenotypes using updated criteria for polycystic ovarian morphology: an assessment of over 100 consecutive women self-reporting features of polycystic ovary syndrome. Reprod Sci 2014;21(8):1034–43.
14. Goodman NF, Cobin RH, Futterweit W, et al. American Association of Clinical Endocrinologists, American College of Endocrinology, and Androgen Excess and PCOS Society Disease State clinical review: guide to the best practices in the evaluation and treatment of polycystic ovary syndrome - part 2. Endocr Pract 2015;21(12):1415–26.
15. Azziz R, Sanchez LA, Knochenhauer ES, et al. Androgen excess in women: experience with over 1000 consecutive patients. J Clin Endocrinol Metab 2004;89(2): 453–62.
16. Lucky AW, McGuire J, Rosenfield RL, et al. Plasma androgens in women with acne vulgaris. J Invest Dermatol 1983;81(1):70–4.
17. Dumesic DA, Lobo RA. Cancer risk and PCOS. Steroids 2013;78(8):782–5.
18. Brassard M, AinMelk Y, Baillargeon JP. Basic infertility including polycystic ovary syndrome. Med Clin North Am 2008;92(5):1163–92, xi.
19. Jakubowicz DJ, Iuorno MJ, Jakubowicz S, et al. Effects of metformin on early pregnancy loss in the polycystic ovary syndrome. J Clin Endocrinol Metab 2002;87(2):524–9.
20. Carmina E, Lobo RA. Use of fasting blood to assess the prevalence of insulin resistance in women with polycystic ovary syndrome. Fertil Steril 2004;82(3): 661–5.
21. Williams T, Mortada R, Porter S. Diagnosis and treatment of polycystic ovary syndrome. Am Fam Physician 2016;94(2):106–13.
22. Woolcock JG, Critchley HO, Munro MG, et al. Review of the confusion in current and historical terminology and definitions for disturbances of menstrual bleeding. Fertil Steril 2008;90(6):2269–80.
23. ACOG Committee on Practice Bulletins–Gynecology. ACOG practice bulletin No. 108: Polycystic ovary syndrome. Obstet Gynecol 2009;114:14.
24. Balen AH, Laven JS, Tan SL, et al. Ultrasound assessment of the polycystic ovary: international consensus definitions. Hum Reprod Update 2003;9(6):505–14.
25. Fauser BC, Tarlatzis BC, Rebar RW, et al. Consensus on women's health aspects of polycystic ovary syndrome (PCOS): the Amsterdam ESHRE/ASRM-sponsored 3rd PCOS Consensus Workshop Group. Fertil Steril 2012;97(1):28–38.e25.

26. Homburg R. The management of infertility associated with polycystic ovary syndrome. Reprod Biol Endocrinol 2003;1:109.
27. Eid GM, Cottam DR, Velcu LM, et al. Effective treatment of polycystic ovarian syndrome with Roux-en-Y gastric bypass. Surg Obes Relat Dis 2005;1(2):77–80.
28. Escobar-Morreale HF, Botella-Carretero JI, Alvarez-Blasco F, et al. The polycystic ovary syndrome associated with morbid obesity may resolve after weight loss induced by bariatric surgery. J Clin Endocrinol Metab 2005;90(12):6364–9.
29. Domecq JP, Prutsky G, Mullan RJ, et al. Lifestyle modification programs in polycystic ovary syndrome: systematic review and meta-analysis. J Clin Endocrinol Metab 2013;98(12):4655–63.
30. Balen AH, Morley LC, Misso M, et al. The management of anovulatory infertility in women with polycystic ovary syndrome: an analysis of the evidence to support the development of global WHO guidance. Hum Reprod Update 2016;22(6): 687–708.
31. Legro RS, Brzyski RG, Diamond MP, et al. The Pregnancy in Polycystic Ovary Syndrome II study: baseline characteristics and effects of obesity from a multicenter randomized clinical trial. Fertil Steril 2014;101(1):258–69.e8.
32. Legro RS, Brzyski RG, Diamond MP, et al. Letrozole versus clomiphene for infertility in the polycystic ovary syndrome. N Engl J Med 2014;371(2):119–29.
33. Tang T, Lord JM, Norman RJ, et al. Insulin-sensitising drugs (metformin, rosiglitazone, pioglitazone, D-chiro-inositol) for women with polycystic ovary syndrome, oligo amenorrhoea and subfertility. Cochrane Database Syst Rev 2012;(5):CD003053.
34. Messinis IE, Milingos SD. Current and future status of ovulation induction in polycystic ovary syndrome. Hum Reprod Update 1997;3(3):235–53.
35. Casper RF, Mitwally MF. Review: aromatase inhibitors for ovulation induction. J Clin Endocrinol Metab 2006;91(3):760–71.
36. Vause TD, Cheung AP, Sierra S, et al. Ovulation induction in polycystic ovary syndrome. J Obstet Gynaecol Can 2010;32(5):495–502.
37. Perales-Puchalt A, Legro RS. Ovulation induction in women with polycystic ovary syndrome. Steroids 2013;78(8):767–72.
38. Thessaloniki ESHRE/ASRM-Sponsored PCOS Consensus Workshop Group. Consensus on infertility treatment related to polycystic ovary syndrome. Fertil Steril 2008;89(3):505–22.
39. Burman ME, Hart AM, Conley V, et al. Reconceptualizing the core of nurse practitioner education and practice. J Am Acad Nurse Pract 2009;21(1):11–7.

Chest Pain

If It Is Not the Heart, What Is It?

Sharron Rushton, DNP, MS, RN, CCM[a],*, Margaret J. Carman, DNP, ACNP-BC, ENP-BC[b]

KEYWORDS

- Noncardiac chest pain • Unexplained chest pain • Angina • Functional chest pain

KEY POINTS

- Noncardiac chest pain can be caused by many etiologies; the priority for management rests in eliminating life-threatening sources first.
- After the differential diagnosis for acute causes of chest pain are eliminated, noncardiac chest pain is differentiated into gastroesophageal reflux disease-related versus non–gastroesophageal reflux disease-related etiologies.
- Patients with noncardiac chest pain can have more than one etiology and may also have a psychological comorbidity.
- Ongoing chest pain from noncardiac chest pain can lead to burden for patients and the health care system.
- Treatment of noncardiac chest pain should be based on management or definitive treatment of the underlying etiology.

INTRODUCTION

A 37-year-old woman with a history of hypertension and obesity presents to her primary care provider for recurrent chest pain that began after going out for breakfast an hour ago. She had a scheduled appointment this morning for follow-up after an overnight stay in the chest pain observation unit over the weekend. An electrocardiogram revealed no acute ischemic changes; serial troponins were within normal limits; an exercise stress test with echocardiography was performed, and the results were negative.

The patient has had recurrent visits to the office and emergency department over the past 6 months. Today's visit is much the same. She describes a tight substernal pressure radiating upward into the base of the throat. She endorses "indigestion,"

Disclosure Statement: The authors have no disclosures of conflict of interest or financial relationships.
[a] Duke University School of Nursing, DUMC Box 3322, Durham, NC 27710, USA; [b] Georgetown University School of Nursing and Health Studies, St. Mary's Hall, 3700 Reservoir Road Northwest, Washington, DC 20007, USA
* Corresponding author.
E-mail address: Sharron.Rushton@duke.edu

Nurs Clin N Am 53 (2018) 421–431
https://doi.org/10.1016/j.cnur.2018.04.009
0029-6465/18/© 2018 Elsevier Inc. All rights reserved.

but denies nausea, vomiting, or abdominal pain. The discomfort makes her anxious, and she is unsure whether that leads to the shortness of breath she is experiencing. The review of systems is otherwise negative.

The nurse practitioner knows this patient fairly well. Given the patient's age and gender, cardiovascular disease seems unlikely. However, her father had his first myocardial infarction at 50 years of age. The patient has a history of smoking history; she quit about 2 years ago. Although it seems reasonable to conclude that a cardiac etiology has been excluded, what could be causing these recurrent episodes of chest pain?

The phenomenon of chest pain can arise from many etiologies but, given the risk of a potentially catastrophic cardiovascular event, it is of utmost importance to diagnose the source of discomfort. Many organs and structures lie within the thoracic cavity, including the cardiac system, vasculature, pulmonary structures, gastroesophageal system, lymphatics, breast, and musculoskeletal components, all of which can cause pain.[1] Pain can be "idiopathic, ischemic, inflammatory, malignant, or related to mechanical disruption from tumor, injury, surgery, or structural failure."[1] Given the numerous structures and disease processes that may manifest as chest pain, it can be difficult to discover the underlying source of the pain.

Noncardiac chest pain (NCCP) is usually described as a burning, angina-like pain located in the sternal area without evidence of ischemic disease.[2–9] NCCP is also known as atypical chest pain, effort syndrome, soldier's heart, irritable heart, DaCosta syndrome, chest pain of unknown origin, neurocirculatory asthenia, cardiac syndrome X, Gorlin-Likoff syndrome, unexplained chest pain, and functional chest pain.[8–11] There are inconsistencies in the literature, especially among various specialties, as to the underlying etiologies and how to classify them. Gastrointestinal specialties consider NCCP to be a unique diagnosis, differentiated as wither gastroesophageal reflux disease (GERD) related or non–GERD related.[7,12,13] Other specialties define NCCP more broadly.[14–18] See **Fig. 1** for a diagram.

The number of conditions contributing to NCCP as well as the various definitions and terms can make it challenging to understand the condition. NCCP occurs in approximately 13% to 25% of the general population and equally in men and

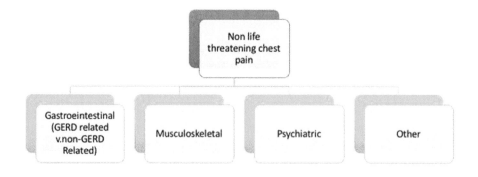

NCCP

Fig. 1. Noncardiac chest pain (NCCP) is classified differently depending on the specialty. The causes are broadly classified into gastrointestinal, musculoskeletal, psychiatric, and pulmonary/other. GERD, gastroesophageal reflux disease.

women.[3,19] However, women are more likely to display anxiety symptoms.[20] Compared with patients who have ischemic chest pain, NCCP patients tend to be younger, have greater anxiety, consume more alcohol, and have higher rates of smoking.[21]

NCCP represents a challenge for the health care system. Chest pain is the second most common cause of emergency room visits.[22,23] NCCP leads to frequent and repeated inpatient or outpatient visits.[11,18,24] For example, the evaluation of nonspecific chest pain accounted for 233,200 emergency department visits in 2011 in patients ages 45 to 64 years.[25] The evaluation of chest pain usually involves intermediate nursing care for electrocardiograms, monitoring, sequential laboratory studies, cardiac stress testing, and various imaging modalities.[26–28]

In addition to the health care system, patients themselves also experience burden. Ongoing chest pain affects these patients' daily lives and results in a decreased quality of life.[7,9–11,29,30] In addition, NCCP can lead to mental strain, employment difficulties, stress at home, and disability.[3,24,29]

ETIOLOGIES OF CHEST PAIN

Life-threatening conditions should be assessed first. Cardiac events that require rapid identification and treatment are not limited to, but include acute coronary syndrome, aortic dissection, aortic stenosis, pericarditis, and pericardial tamponade.[3,31–34] Extracardiac conditions could include tension pneumothorax, pulmonary embolism, or esophageal rupture.[3,31–34]

The nurse practitioner feels a bit reassured after eliciting an updated history from the patient. It seems that she has had increasing stress at work over the past year that align to when episodes began. The pain is often associated with eating a large meal after she's worked all day without a break. She's been living on coffee to keep her going and has taken a second job to make ends meet. Often, she will try to get to sleep after grabbing some food late at night, and that's when the pain sets in. Could it be attributed to GERD? Stress?

Some forms of NCCP will have a specific underlying condition and some have traits similar to other unexplained physical symptoms.[14] Three primary categories of NCCP have been identified including musculoskeletal, upper gastrointestinal and those with a psychological component.[8,10,35]

- Gastrointestinal disorders that can cause chest pain are generally traced to the esophagus, hypersensitivities, or motor disorders.[3,36,37] Of the gastrointestinal disorders, GERD is the most likely cause of NCCP.[3,36,38]
- Musculoskeletal chest wall pain can arise from conditions leading to isolated pain, rheumatic disease, or other systemic diseases.[39] Costochondritis is most often the cause of musculoskeletal chest pain.[40]
- Psychological disorders such as anxiety and depression may also lead to chest pain.[6,41] Panic attacks may also play a role in NCCP.[9]

A sampling of potential etiologies can be found in **Fig. 2**.

Given the complexity of NCCP, the pathophysiology underlying NCCP has not been clearly defined. This is in part due to the vast number of conditions that can cause NCCP, leading to potentially multiple mechanisms. For example, gastroesophageal NCCP could be secondary to refluxate, changes in receptors, or alterations in the sensing or processing of neural stimuli.[42–44] In addition, patients with NCCP may display abnormal thoracic breathing (hyperventilation).[45] To add to the complexity, patients may also present with more than 1 physiologic cause. Husser and associates[17]

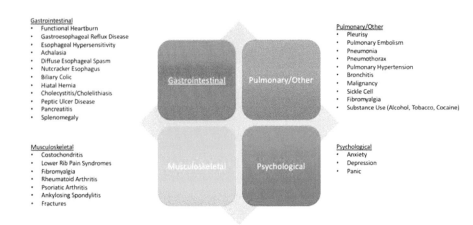

Gastrointestinal
- Functional Heartburn
- Gastroesophageal Reflux Disease
- Esophageal Hypersensitivity
- Achalasia
- Diffuse Esophageal Spasm
- Nutcracker Esophagus
- Biliary Colic
- Hiatal Hernia
- Cholecystitis/Cholelithiasis
- Peptic Ulcer Disease
- Pancreatitis
- Splenomegaly

Musculoskeletal
- Costochondritis
- Lower Rib Pain Syndromes
- Fibromyalgia
- Rheumatoid Arthritis
- Psoriatic Arthritis
- Ankylosing Spondylitis
- Fractures

Pulmonary/Other
- Pleurisy
- Pulmonary Embolism
- Pneumonia
- Pneumothorax
- Pulmonary Hypertension
- Bronchitis
- Malignancy
- Sickle Cell
- Fibromyalgia
- Substance Use (Alcohol, Tobacco, Cocaine)

Psychological
- Anxiety
- Depression
- Panic

Fig. 2. Examples of the differential for a chief complaint of chest pain.

reviewed the noncardiac causes of chest pain in 37 patients and found that approximately 16% of patients had more than 1 diagnosis. As another example, fibromyalgia has been associated with NCCP.[46]

Psychological conditions were noted elsewhere in this article to be a potential etiology. A psychological condition may be co-present with NCCP in some patients.[3,43,44] Patients with NCCP may have a combination of psychiatric conditions and asthma, pneumonia, musculoskeletal, or other painful conditions.[7,16,47] Depression and anxiety specifically have been associated with NCCP and can impact pain.[3,47] In addition, NCCP patient tend to do more self-monitoring and had poorer coping skills.[48,49]

Lifestyle choices also potentially lead to the development of chest pain that requires investigating cardiac versus noncardiac sources. Food choices such as greasy/rich foods, spicy foods, acidic foods such as tomatoes and citrus fruits, peppermint, and overeating are considered risk factors for NCCP.[9,10] Drinks such as alcohol and carbonated beverages are also risk factors.[10] In addition to smoking being a risk factor for coronary artery disease, it is potentially a risk factor for GERD.[10,33,50,51] There is also relationship between anxiety and smoking.[52] Cocaine can lead to chest pain owing to its impact on the sympathetic nervous system, myocytes, and vasculature.[35,53]

PEDIATRICS

Although this article focuses on adults, children also experience chest pain. Noncardiac causes are the most common cause of chest pain in children, and occur in about 56% to 86% of cases in children.[54,55] Children under 12 years of age are more likely to have cardiopulmonary causes, whereas teenagers are more likely to have other underlying causes.[56] The average age of presentation in children is the early teens.[54] Pain that is chronic is more commonly associated with noncardiac causes, but the cause can be difficult to find.[54,55] Sources for NCCP in children include idiopathic, musculoskeletal, pulmonary, psychiatric, and gastrointestinal.[54,56,57] Children may also have more than 1 contributing factor.[56] Referral to pediatric cardiology would be recommended for red flags, such as a concerning history or abnormal workup, and an emergency workup for acute onset with fever.[55] NCCP should also be considered in children who experience abuse because they have an increased risk for this condition.[58]

ASSESSMENT

Although the first course of action should be to rule out those conditions that threaten life and limb, Morrow[31] outlines an approach to consider after the urgent, life-threatening diagnoses have been excluded: (1) Did a complication of a chronic disease lead to the pain? (2) Did an acute condition give rise to the pain? (3) Is the pain secondary to another condition? Given the numerous differentials involved in a patient who presents with chest pain, it is impossible for all potential workups to be reviewed, so GERD, costochondritis, and anxiety are used as exemplars for underlying the etiologies of NCCP.

Taking a thorough history should provide information about the chest pain specifics.[35,59,60] There are multiple methods for assessing pain. For example, pain can be assessed using OPQRST (onset/chronology, provocative or palliative, quality of symptoms, region or area, severity, temporal pattern).[60–62] Another example includes OLDCARTS (onset, location, duration, characteristics, aggravating, relieving factors, and treatment or temporal).[63] There are several pain assessment tools available as well, such as the McGill Pain Assessment Questionnaire, numeric rating scales, or visual analog scales.[63] Associated symptoms should also be considered such as nausea, diaphoresis, dyspnea, neurologic symptoms, or palpitations.[60] In addition to pain, a review of systems includes chief complaint, history of the present illness, history (past medical, family, personal, social), perceived health status, functional status, medication use, and substance use.[27] Suggested body systems to include in the review of systems and physical examination can be found in **Fig. 3**.

After cardiovascular disorders are ruled out, gastroesophageal conditions, primarily GERD, may be considered if the pain is associated with dysphagia, heartburn, and/or odynophagia in combination with an achy feeling that lasts for at least 1 hour.[33,35,37] Additional symptoms may include pain associated with a meal and a nonsmoker's cough that lasts more than 3 weeks.[32,64] The GerdQ and Reflux Disease Questionnaire are tools that can be used to evaluate for GERD.[64,65] Clinical history is not generally enough, and additional testing should be considered.[66] Some have advocated first diagnostic approach by a proton pump inhibitor (PPI) trial if an esophageal cause is suspected.[2,12,67] The evaluation of symptoms may suggest red flags such as anemia,

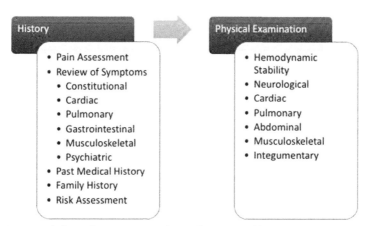

Fig. 3. History and physical examination. The performance of history and physical are important to the diagnosis of noncardiac chest pain. The presentation of the patient will guide both, but body systems to consider are denoted.

loss of appetite, dysphagia, unintentional weight loss, odynophagia, or hematemesis for which an upper endoscopy will likely be completed.[12,36,64,67] If the results of PPI trial and/or endoscopy do not yield sufficient results then additional testing such as wireless pH capsule may be considered.[68]

Chest pain that is reproducible with movement such as manipulation or palpation, with supporting evidence such as trauma or infection, is suggestive of a musculoskeletal etiology.[32,35,59,69] Costochondritis can be described as achy, pressure-like or sharp pain that which may be aggravated with deep breathing or motion and is best evaluated with radiographs, a computed tomography scan, or bone scan.[33,40]

Psychiatric conditions such as anxiety may lead to NCCP. Patients who complain of acute coronary syndrome type symptoms lasting at least half an hour may be experiencing anxiety or a panic attack.[28,33] Psychological assessment should include knowledge and perceptions of the cause for their chest pain, and adherence to treatment. Psychological risk factors should be considered, as well as a functional behavioral analysis and behavioral reactions to pain.[70] Evidence-based care includes the use of screening and assessment instruments.[70,71] The workup should be based on signs and symptoms, laboratory tests and imaging studies as well as the use of assessment tools which may include: Generalized Anxiety Disorder (GAD) 2, Generalized Anxiety Disorder (GAD) 7, and/or the Hospital Anxiety and Depression Scale.[71–74]

The nurse practitioner consults with the cardiologist who performed the stress study on the patient. Given the negative workup, cardiac etiologies are ruled out. The patient's examination does not indicate pulmonary or musculoskeletal abnormalities. The nurse practitioner begins a course of omeprazole and makes a referral to gastroenterology for probable endoscopy. The patient's complete blood count and chemistries are within normal limits. There is low risk for thromboembolism or infectious etiology. The next step in formalizing a diagnosis will be to differentiate whether her pain is related to esophageal reflux.

TREATMENT CONSIDERATIONS

There is no specific treatment for NCCP; instead, treatment is aimed at the identified etiology. The workup of NCCP is therefore critical for optimal treatment.[35] It is not possible within the scope of this article to discuss all possible treatment options, so the same exemplars will be used.

- GERD treatment begins with lifestyle and behavioral modifications. Weight loss, avoidance of food triggers, and elevating the head of bed are recommended.[67] Tobacco can also aggravate symptoms of GERD-related NCCP, so working with the patient on smoking cessation is also of value.[26] The American College of Gastroenterology guidelines and others recommend treating GERD-related NCCP with PPI therapy.[4,37,67] Additional therapies depend on PPI response.[67,68]
- Costochondritis can resolve on its own.[69,75] Additional treatment for costochondritis includes rest, reassurance, nonnarcotic pain control, nonpharmacologic pain management (ice or heat), and stretching.[40,69]
- Generalized anxiety can be treated with certain antidepressants followed by other anxiolytics.[71,76] Patients with NCCP of a psychiatric nature may benefit from reassurance about their prognosis in addition to cognitive therapy, biopsychosocial model, hypnotherapy, and biofeedback.[36,77,78]

Addressing the psychological impact of ongoing chest pain and psychological comorbidities are important because patients tend to experience decreased quality of life and psychological distress.[14,30,68] Treatment should be individualized to address a patient's needs because this measure results in better adherence, improved coping, and successful treatment.[70] As an example, patients may not fully understand their ongoing chest pain and want more information.[79] Thus, an intervention aimed to improve knowledge as well as strategies to address pain and stress could be useful as well as one that includes a psychiatric referral.[78,80] Patients with NCCP may also benefit from cognitive-behavioral therapy.[4,7,81] Chambers and colleagues[14] recommend using the biopsychosocial model for treatment, which includes supporting the patient with explanations and reassurance, connecting him or her with social resources, administering medication based on clinical indication, teaching relaxation methods, and making referrals to specialists as needed. The biopsychosocial approach was able to decrease the number of chest pain episodes, decrease activity avoidance, improve psychological distress, and reduce health care use and work absences related to chest pain.[45]

The patient returns to clinic 6 weeks later for a follow-up. She notes that the constant burning has improved, but she continues to have episodic chest tightness with sweating. She now reports to the provider that she lost her mom to cancer about 3 months ago, and endorses feeling lost and anxious. The patient and provider decide that she should follow up with psychiatry for a full evaluation.

SUMMARY

For health care providers, NCCP is a challenging disorder given it heterogeneous nature. The term NCCP is generally understood to mean angina without evidence of ischemia, but there is there is lack of consensus of other aspects among the specialties. The lack of understanding of the pathophysiology and the coexistence of multiple etiologies in some patients adds to the complexity. Comprehensive evaluation is often insufficient for diagnosis or identification of an underlying etiology. Treatment can be complex requiring addressing multiple factors such as comorbidities and psychosocial factors.

From the patient's perspective, the experience of having chest pain can be frightening. Ongoing chest pain can prompt dramatic alterations to daily life and ongoing interactions with the health care system. NCCP can have financial implications and decreased quality of life. It is crucial that the health care provider have an appreciation for the impact of NCCP on patients' well-being, even when it is not the result of a life-threatening condition.

REFERENCES

1. Gottschalk A, Ochroch EA. Thoracic pain. In: McMahon SB, Koltzenburg M, Tracey I, et al, editors. Wall & Melzack's textbook of pain. 6th edition. Philadelphia: Elsevier Saunders; 2013. p. 718–33.
2. Coss-Adame E, Rao SS. A review of esophageal chest pain. Gastroenterol Hepatol 2015;11(11):759–66.
3. Fass R, Achem SR. Noncardiac chest pain: epidemiology, natural course and pathogenesis. J Neurogastroenterol Motil 2011;17(2):110–23.
4. Hershcovici T, Achem SR, Jha LK, et al. Systematic review: the treatment of noncardiac chest pain. Aliment Pharmacol Ther 2012;35(1):5–14.
5. Leise MD, Locke GR 3rd, Dierkhising RA, et al. Patients dismissed from the hospital with a diagnosis of noncardiac chest pain: cardiac outcomes and health care utilization. Mayo Clin Proc 2010;85(4):323–30.
6. Lenfant C. Chest pain of cardiac and noncardiac origin. Metabolism 2010; 59(Suppl 1):S41–6.

7. Schey R, Villarreal A, Fass R. Noncardiac chest pain: current treatment. Gastroenterol Hepatol 2007;3(4):255–62.
8. Chambers JB, Marks EM, Hunter MS. The head says yes but the heart says no: what is non-cardiac chest pain and how is it managed? Heart 2015;101(15): 1240–9.
9. Eslick GD. Noncardiac chest pain: epidemiology, natural history, health care seeking, and quality of life. Gastroenterol Clin North Am 2004;33(1):1–23.
10. Eslick GD. Classification, natural history, epidemiology, and risk factors of noncardiac chest pain. Dis Mon 2008;54(9):593–603.
11. Roll M, Rosenqvist M, Sjoborg B, et al. Unexplained acute chest pain in young adults: disease patterns and medication use 25 years later. Psychosom Med 2015;77(5):567–74.
12. Fass R. Evaluation and diagnosis of noncardiac chest pain. Dis Mon 2008;54(9): 627–41.
13. Gill RS, Collins JS, Talley NJ. Management of noncardiac chest pain in women. Womens Health (Lond) 2012;8(2):131–43 [quiz: 144–5].
14. Chambers JB, Marks E, Knisley L, et al. Non-cardiac chest pain: time to extend the rapid access chest pain clinic? Int J Clin Pract 2013;67(4):303–6.
15. Yelland M, Cayley WE Jr, Vach W. An algorithm for the diagnosis and management of chest pain in primary care. Med Clin North Am 2010;94(2):349–74.
16. Ruigomez A, Masso-Gonzalez EL, Johansson S, et al. Chest pain without established ischaemic heart disease in primary care patients: associated comorbidities and mortality. Br J Gen Pract 2009;59(560):e78–86.
17. Husser D, Bollmann A, Kuhne C, et al. Evaluation of noncardiac chest pain: diagnostic approach, coping strategies and quality of life. Eur J Pain 2006;10(1):51–5.
18. Safdar B, Dziura J, Bathulapalli H, et al. Chest pain syndromes are associated with high rates of recidivism and costs in young United States Veterans. BMC Fam Pract 2015;16:88.
19. Ford AC, Suares NC, Talley NJ. Meta-analysis: the epidemiology of noncardiac chest pain in the community. Aliment Pharmacol Ther 2011;34(2):172–80.
20. Carmin CN, Ownby RL, Wiegartz PS, et al. Women and non-cardiac chest pain: gender differences in symptom presentation. Arch Womens Ment Health 2008; 11(4):287–93.
21. Tew R, Guthrie EA, Creed FH, et al. A long-term follow-up study of patients with ischaemic heart disease versus patients with nonspecific chest pain. J Psychosom Res 1995;39(8):977–85.
22. Strehlow M, Tabas J. Chest pain. In: Adams JG, editor. Emergency medicine,. 2nd edition. Philadelphia: Elsevier, Saunders; 2013. p. 445–51.e441.
23. Skinner HG, Blanchard J, Elixhauser A. Trends in emergency department visits, 2006-2011: statistical brief #179. Healthcare cost and utilization project (HCUP) statistical briefs. Rockville (MD): Agency for healthcare research and quality (US); 2006.
24. Chambers J, Bass C. Chest pain with normal coronary anatomy: a review of natural history and possible etiologic factors. Prog Cardiovasc Dis 1990;33(3): 161–84.
25. Weiss AJ, Wier LM, Stocks C, et al. Overview of emergency department visits in the United States. Rockville (MD): Healthcare Cost and Utilization Project: Agency for Healthcare Research and Quality; 2014. p. 1–13.
26. Ignatavicius DD, Workman ML. Care of patients with esophageal problems. In: Medical surgical nursing: patient-centered collaborative care. 7th edition. St Louis (MO): Elsevier.; 2013. p. 1205–8.

27. Levine BS. History taking and physical examination. In: Woods SL, Froelicher ESS, Motzer SA, editors. Cardiac nursing. Philadelphia: Lippincott Williams & Wilkins; 2010. p. 211–44.

28. Sabatine MS, Cannon CP. Approach to the patient with chest pain. In: Mann DL, Zipes DP, Libby P, et al, editors. Braunwald's heart disease: a textbook of cardiovascular medicine, vol. 50, 10th edition. Philadelphia: Elsevier, Saunders; 2015. p. 1057–67.

29. Jerlock M, Kjellgren KI, Gaston-Johansson F, et al. Psychosocial profile in men and women with unexplained chest pain. J Intern Med 2008;264(3):265–74.

30. Webster R, Norman P, Goodacre S, et al. Illness representations, psychological distress and non-cardiac chest pain in patients attending an emergency department. Psychol Health 2014;29(11):1265–82.

31. Morrow DA. Chest discomfort. In: Kasper D, Fauci A, Hauser S, et al, editors. Harrison's Principles of Internal Medicine. 19th edition. New York: McGraw-Hill Education; 2015.

32. Runion SE, Lamb EM. Quick guide to rule out chest pain emergencies. Am J Nurse Pract 2007;11(6):21–31.

33. Baas AS, Huang DT. Chest pain. In: Vincent J-L, Abraham E, Moore FA, et al, editors. Textbook of critical care. 7th edition. Philadelphia: Elsevier; 2017. p. 123–7.e1.

34. Brown JE. Chest pain. In: Walls RM, Hockberger RS, Gausche-Hill M, editors. Rosen's emergency medicine: concepts and clinical practice. 9th edition. Philadelphia: Elsevier; 2018. p. 204–12.

35. Fenster BE, Lee-Chiong TL, Gebhart GF, et al. Chest pain. In: Broaddus VC, Mason RJ, Ernst JD, et al, editors. Murray and Nadel's textbook of respiratory medicine. 6th edition. Philadelphia: Elsevier, Saunders; 2016. p. 515–26.e3.

36. Arora AS, Katzka DA. How do I handle the patient with noncardiac chest pain? Clin Gastroenterol Hepatol 2011;9(4):295–304 [quiz: e35].

37. Oranu AC, Vaezi MF. Noncardiac chest pain: gastroesophageal reflux disease. Med Clin North Am 2010;94(2):233–42.

38. Fass R, Navarro-Rodriguez T. Noncardiac chest pain. J Clin Gastroenterol 2008; 42(5):636–46.

39. Winzenberg T, Jones G, Callisaya M. Musculoskeletal chest wall pain. Aust Fam Physician 2015;44(8):540–4.

40. Ayloo A, Cvengros T, Marella S. Evaluation and treatment of musculoskeletal chest pain. Prim Care 2013;40(4):863–87, viii.

41. Eken C, Oktay C, Bacanli A, et al. Anxiety and depressive disorders in patients presenting with chest pain to the emergency department: a comparison between cardiac and non-cardiac origin. J Emerg Med 2010;39(2):144–50.

42. Aziz Q, Fass R, Gyawali CP, et al. Functional esophageal disorders. Gastroenterology 2016;150(6):1368–79.

43. Van Handel D, Fass R. The pathophysiology of non-cardiac chest pain. J Gastroenterol Hepatol 2005;20(Suppl):S6–13.

44. Kindt S, Tack J. Pathophysiology of noncardiac chest pain: not only acid. Dis Mon 2008;54(9):615–26.

45. Chambers JB, Marks EM, Russell V, et al. A multidisciplinary, biopsychosocial treatment for non-cardiac chest pain. Int J Clin Pract 2015;69(9):922–7.

46. Almansa C, Wang B, Achem SR. Noncardiac chest pain and fibromyalgia. Med Clin North Am 2010;94(2):275–89.

47. Smeijers L, van de Pas H, Nyklicek I, et al. The independent association of anxiety with non-cardiac chest pain. Psychol Health 2014;29(3):253–63.

48. Cheng C, Wong WM, Lai KC, et al. Psychosocial factors in patients with noncardiac chest pain. Psychosom Med 2003;65(3):443–9.

49. White KS, Craft JM, Gervino EV. Anxiety and hypervigilance to cardiopulmonary sensations in non-cardiac chest pain patients with and without psychiatric disorders. Behav Res Ther 2010;48(5):394–401.

50. Al Talalwah N, Woodward S. Gastro-oesophageal reflux. Part 1: smoking and alcohol reduction. Br J Nurs 2013;22(3):140–2, 144–6.

51. Hallan A, Bomme M, Hveem K, et al. Risk factors on the development of new-onset gastroesophageal reflux symptoms. A population-based prospective cohort study: the HUNT study. Am J Gastroenterol 2015;110(3):393–400 [quiz: 401].

52. Jiang F, Li S, Pan L, et al. Association of anxiety disorders with the risk of smoking behaviors: a meta-analysis of prospective observational studies. Drug Alcohol Depend 2014;145:69–76.

53. Stankowski RV, Kloner RA, Rezkalla SH. Cardiovascular consequences of cocaine use. Trends Cardiovasc Med 2015;25(6):517–26.

54. Park MK. Child with chest pain. In: Park MK, editor. Park's pediatric cardiology for practitioners. Philadelphia: Elsevier Saunders; 2014. p. 495–504.

55. Yeh TK, Yeh J. Chest pain in pediatrics. Pediatr Ann 2015;44(12):e274–8.

56. Kolinski JM. Chest pain. In: Kliegman RM, Lye PS, Bordini BJ, et al, editors. Nelson pediatric symptom-based diagnosis. Philadelphia: Elsevier; 2018. p. 104–15.e1.

57. Kim YJ, Shin EJ, Kim NS, et al. The importance of esophageal and gastric diseases as causes of chest pain. Pediatr Gastroenterol Hepatol Nutr 2015;18(4): 261–7.

58. Eslick GD, Koloski NA, Talley NJ. Sexual, physical, verbal/emotional abuse and unexplained chest pain. Child Abuse Negl 2011;35(8):601–5.

59. Cayley WE Jr. Diagnosing the cause of chest pain. Am Fam Physician 2005; 72(10):2012–21.

60. Reigle J. Evaluating the patient with chest pain: the value of a comprehensive history. J Cardiovasc Nurs 2005;20(4):226–31.

61. Ball JW, Dains JE, Flynn JA, et al. Vital signs and pain assessment. In: Seidel's guide to physical examination. 8th edition. St Louis (MO): Elsevier, Mosby; 2015. p. 50–63.

62. Swartz M. The interviewers questions. In: Swartz M, editor. Textbook of physical diagnosis. 7th edition. Philadelphia: Elsevier, Saunders; 2014. p. 3–39.e3.

63. DAmico D, Barbarito C. Pain assessment. Health & physical assessment in nursing. 2nd edition. Boston (MA): Pearson; 2011.

64. Anderson WD 3rd, Strayer SM, Mull SR. Common questions about the management of gastroesophageal reflux disease. Am Fam Physician 2015;91(10):692–7.

65. Bolier EA, Kessing BF, Smout AJ, et al. Systematic review: questionnaires for assessment of gastroesophageal reflux disease. Dis Esophagus 2015;28(2): 105–20.

66. Jerlock M, Welin C, Rosengren A, et al. Pain characteristics in patients with unexplained chest pain and patients with ischemic heart disease. Eur J Cardiovasc Nurs 2007;6(2):130–6.

67. Katz PO, Gerson LB, Vela MF. Guidelines for the diagnosis and management of gastroesophageal reflux disease. Am J Gastroenterol 2013;108(3):308–28 [quiz: 329].

68. Yamasaki T, Fass R. Noncardiac chest pain: diagnosis and management. Curr Opin Gastroenterol 2017;33(4):293–300.

69. Stochkendahl MJ, Christensen HW. Chest pain in focal musculoskeletal disorders. Med Clin North Am 2010;94(2):259–73.
70. White KS. Assessment and treatment of psychological causes of chest pain. Med Clin North Am 2010;94(2):291–318.
71. Rothberg B, Schneck CD. Anxiety and depression. In: Rakel RE, Rakel DP, editors. Textbook of family medicine,. 9th edition. Philadelphia: Elsevier, Saunders; 2016. p. 1090–107.e3.
72. Plummer F, Manea L, Trepel D, et al. Screening for anxiety disorders with the GAD-7 and GAD-2: a systematic review and diagnostic metaanalysis. Gen Hosp Psychiatry 2016;39:24–31.
73. Zigmond AS, Snaith RP. The hospital anxiety and depression scale. Acta Psychiatr Scand 1983;67(6):361–70.
74. Dalrymple KL. Anxiety (Generalized Anxiety Disorder). In: Ferri F, editor. Ferri's clinical advisor 2018. Philadelphia: Elsevier; 2018. p. 110.
75. Shrestha A. Costochondritis. In: Ferri G, editor. Ferri's clinical advisor 2018. Philadelphia: Elsevier; 2018. p. 343–343.e341.
76. Rang HP, Ritter JM, Flower RJ, et al. Anxiolytic and hypnotic drugs. Rang and Dale's pharmacology. 8th edition. London (United Kingdom): Elsevier Churchill Livingstone; 2016. p. 536–45.
77. Achem SR. Noncardiac chest pain-treatment approaches. Gastroenterol Clin North Am 2008;37(4):859–78, ix.
78. Kisely SR, Campbell LA, Yelland MJ, et al. Psychological interventions for symptomatic management of non-specific chest pain in patients with normal coronary anatomy. Cochrane Database Syst Rev 2015;(6):CD004101.
79. Roysland IO, Dysvik E, Furnes B, et al. Exploring the information needs of patients with unexplained chest pain. Patient Prefer Adherence 2013;7:915–23.
80. Webster R, Thompson AR, Norman P. 'Everything's fine, so why does it happen?' A qualitative investigation of patients' perceptions of noncardiac chest pain. J Clin Nurs 2015;24(13–14):1936–45.
81. George N, Abdallah J, Maradey-Romero C, et al. Review article: the current treatment of non-cardiac chest pain. Aliment Pharmacol Ther 2016;43(2):213–39.

Evaluation and Treatment of Restless Legs Syndrome in the Primary Care Environment

Benjamin A. Smallheer, PhD, RN, ACNP-BC, FNP-BC, CCRN, CNE

KEYWORDS

- Restless legs syndrome • Primary care • Willis-Ekbon disease • Evaluation
- Treatment

KEY POINTS

- Restless legs syndrome/Willis-Ekbon disease (RLS/WED) is a common sensorimotor disorder characterized by an urge to move.
- RLS/WED is associated with an uncomfortable sensation typically in the lower extremities.
- Iron deficiency, dopaminergic neurotransmission abnormalities, genetics, sleep deprivation, immobilization, and/or use of medications can play key roles in the pathogenesis of primary (idiopathic) RLS.
- Identification and treatment through a thorough subjective evaluation and complete neurologic examination are essential in the diagnosis of RLS/WED.
- Dopaminergic agents and alpha-2-delta calcium channel ligands are the more common and effective pharmacologic agents used to treat RLS.

INTRODUCTION

Restless legs syndrome (RLS) is a common neurologic sensorimotor disorder characterized by an irresistible urge to move the legs repetitively. Also referred to as Willis-Ekbom disease (WED), this syndrome has undergone increasing research over the past decade; there is now a more complete understanding of its cause, diagnostic criteria, and treatment algorithms.

The Diagnostic Classification of Sleep and Arousal Disorders, produced by the International Restless Legs Syndrome Study Group (IRLSSG), classified RLS/WED as a disorder of initiating and maintaining sleep and of excessive somnolence. Individuals experience "extremely disagreeable deep sensations of creeping inside the calves whenever sitting or lying down."[1] This sleep-related disorder of movement is associated with discomfort and dysesthesia, occurs more during periods of inactivity (ie, at night), and, thus, interferes with sleep.

Duke University School of Nursing, 307 Trent Drive, DUMC Box 3322, Durham, NC 27710, USA
E-mail address: benjamin.smallheer@duke.edu

Nurs Clin N Am 53 (2018) 433–445
https://doi.org/10.1016/j.cnur.2018.04.010
0029-6465/18/© 2018 Elsevier Inc. All rights reserved.

RLS is typically described as a nocturnal disorder based on its profound distur-bance of sleep.[2,3] As a result, this circadian disturbance has been shown to have a cascading impact on both physiologic and psychological health, ultimately affecting mood and quality of life.[1,3]

PREVALENCE, EPIDEMIOLOGY, AND CAUSE

In 1672, English physician and anatomist Sir Thomas Willis became the first to describe RLS.[4,5] Later, in 1763, symptoms comparable with RLS were described by French physician and botanist François Boissier de Sauvages, in 1849 by Swedish physician and professor Magnus Huss, and in 1898 by French physician Georges Gilles de la Tourette.[4] The term restless legs syndrome was introduced in 1945 by the Swedish neurologist Karl Axel Ekbom, who conducted the first clinical and epidemiologic studies on the topic. In 1995, the IRLSSG devel-oped the initial RLS standardized diagnostic criteria, which have since been updated.[4,5]

RLS/WED affects 5% to 15% of adults in the United States and Northern Europe, with a higher prevalence in women than men at a ratio of almost 2:1. This increased risk in women is thought to be related to parity, as the incidence in nulliparous women is similar to the incidence seen in men. Women who have been pregnant have a 2 times increased risk for developing RLS compared with nulliparous women. During pregnancy, RLS/WED has been identified in 13.5% to 26.6% of pregnant woman. It tends to develop more frequently during the third trimester but becomes more severe over the duration of the pregnancy.[3,6] Additionally, women who have experienced transient RLS during pregnancy have a 4 times increased risk for developing persis-tent RLS over the life course.[1,2,7-9]

The incidence of RLS in children occurs in 2% to 4% of school-aged children and adolescents. Of these children, symptoms range from mild to severe, with 25% to 50% of children reporting moderate to severe symptoms. Predictably, the incidence is higher among children whereby a family history reveals parents with RLS.[2,7]

RLS has been shown to occur less frequently in African Americans compared with Caucasians despite all other confounding risk factors.[8] More developed research has shown that, in addition to affecting the lower extremities, RLS/WED has also been re-ported to affect the arms.[3] RLS is traditionally considered a chronic, lifelong disease that worsens with time. Periods of remission are common, especially in younger adults; relapse is not uncommon or unexpected.[1,3,10] These various presentations of RLS have been known to fluctuate depending on the cause of the syndrome. For example, incidents associated with pregnancy often disappear within the first month following delivery.[6] Additionally, occurrences of RLS/WED associated with other reversible causes, such as iron deficiencies or uremia, may diminish following correc-tion of the causative factors.

SYMPTOM PRESENTATION

Individuals use a variety of terms to describe the sensations associated with RLS/WED. Dysesthesia sensations are typically relieved by movement, exacerbated by rest or inactivity, and worse in the evening/night.[10] Symptoms are often associated with paresthesias. **Box 1** lists the more common symptoms reported by patients living with RLS/WED.

RLS/WED is commonly associated with the disorder known as periodic limb move-ments of sleep (PLMS), which is described as involuntary and repetitive cramping and jerking movements of the legs. The presence of periodic limb movements during sleep

---

Box 1
Symptoms experienced by patients living with restless legs syndrome/Willis-Ekbom disease

- Aching
- Bubbling
- Burning
- Creepy-crawly
- Electric current sensations
- Fidgeting
- Itching
- Jittering
- Pressure
- Pulling/drawing up
- Tightness
- Tingling
- Throbbing
- Worms or insects moving

Data from Refs.[2,3,8]

---

is experienced at greater rates and intensity than expected for a patient's age or medical/medication status.[1] The urge to move is similar to RLS/WED in that it is worse during rest and at night, leading to sleep disruption. It occurs approximately every 20 to 40 seconds. Although often associated with RLS, the condition is not the same and has a separate diagnosis. The differentiation lies in that PLMS affects individuals only while they are asleep, whereas RLS/WED affects individuals while at rest but awake. Individuals with RLS often concomitantly report having PLMS, but individuals with PLMS do not necessarily experience the awake symptoms of RLS. PLMS and RLS/WED are distinct, mutually exclusive diagnoses and may or may not be associated with arousal from sleep.[5,11,12]

When operationalizing RLS/WED, patients may experience symptoms at varying frequencies. Symptoms may occur at frequencies less than once a year to multiple times daily. Daily symptoms have been found to affect middle-aged individuals in a progressive clinical manner and are less frequently reported in clients less than 40 to 60 years of age.[1,3,10,13] Severity of symptoms may remit for various periods of time and may fluctuate from extremely mild and of no significance to the patients' routine to a level of annoyance that is extremely disabling. It is at this level of extreme disability that patients often report substantial sleep disturbances and an impact on quality of life.[1,2] This impact on quality of life of RLS/WED has been shown to be as significant as major medical diagnoses, such as diabetes mellitus type 2 and osteoarthritis.[3]

CAUSES OF AND ASSOCIATIONS WITH RESTLESS LEGS SYNDROME/WILLIS-EKBON DISEASE

Causes and associations of RLS/WED have been moderately researched in the past decade. Of significance, it has been discovered that RLS is more common in patients with chronic kidney disease, iron deficiency anemia, pregnancy, diabetes, neuropathy, and chronic neurologic disorders. The relationship with iron deficiency, pregnancy, uremia, and neurologic problems, although idiopathic, have been observed to have greater associations in clinical research to RLS/WED than other known causes.[1,3] Within the pediatric population, current evidence supports relative iron deficiency and renal failure as potential and prominent aggravating factors.[14] Other diseases that have recognized and significant associations with RLS/WED can be found in **Box 2**.

RLS seems to follow a pattern of autosomal dominant inheritance, although occurrences without any genetic links are also found.[8] The dissemination of this disorder has variable expressions not only influenced by genetics but also influenced by both environmental and medical factors.[1] The genetic component of autosomal dominance together with age-dependent prevalence, a dopaminergic receptor functionality, and iron metabolism dysregulation play an important role in the development of repetitive, nonepileptiform movements of the lower limbs, which is the signature physiologic characteristic of RLS.[13,15] Additional studies associating animal models with human models have shown that increased tyrosine hydroxylase concentrations in the substantia nigra, which directly influence enzymes associated with dopamine synthesis, have been shown to directly decrease the number of D_2 dopamine receptors and increase the concentrations of specific dopamine receptors in the brain. This

---

Box 2
Medical diagnosis associated with restless legs syndrome/Willis-Ekbom disease

- Adults greater than 45 years of age
- Cardiovascular disease
- Cerebellar ataxia
- Charcot-Marie-Tooth disease (type 2)
- Dementia
- Diabetes mellitus
- Fibromyalgia
- Multiple sclerosis
- Narcolepsy
- Obesity
- Obstructive sleep apnea
- Rheumatologic disorders
- Parkinson disease
- Peripheral neuropathy
- Radiculopathy
- Renal disease (chronic and end stage)
- Rheumatoid arthritis
- Spinal cord lesions
- Spinal nerve root irritation
- Spinocerebellar ataxia

Data from Refs.[1-3,13]

finding implies that the syndrome is characterized by the upregulation of dopaminergic transmission and postsynaptic desensitization.[3]

RLS can be categorized into either a primary (idiopathic) or secondary disease. Most primary cases have an unknown origin, thereby earning the nomenclature of idiopathic RLS/WED.[13] Early research suggests possible associations between idiopathic RLS/WED and dopaminergic system dysfunction, brain iron metabolism, neurotransmitter alterations, and inflammatory and immune mechanisms. A strong genetic component does seem to exist, especially among first-degree relatives.[1] A widely significant genetic variance of 18.5% to 59.6% has been found to influence an individual's risk of developing RLS/WED.[3] Six different genes have been identified as significant to the development and progression of RLS/WED. These genes are *BTBD9, MEIS1, PTPRD, MAP2K5, SKOR1,* and *TOX3*.[3,13] These genes play a vital role, along with the impact of both dopaminergic reception and brain iron dysregulation. Extensive genome association studies have shown these associations have also been associated with PLMS disorders. The role each of these genes plays remains unclear, and specific causes for these associations have yet to be identified.

Unlike primary (idiopathic) RLS, which does not have a clear or recognized cause, secondary RLS occurs as a result of certain conditions. Secondary RLS tends to appear in later life and occurs in the presence of other complex medical conditions, often making diagnosis more challenging. The presence of other neurologic conditions that might mimic RLS symptoms, such as Parkinson disease, attention-deficit/ hyperactive disorder, fibromyalgia, meralgia paresthetica, drug-induced dyskinesias, and peripheral neuropathies from a host of pathologies, can cause a delay in the timely diagnosis and treatment of RLS.[3,7,16] Within the pediatric population, common mimicking conditions are more often associated with injury. Common conditions include the following:

- Bruises
- Dermatitis
- Growing pains
- Ligament and/or tendon sprain
- Positional discomfort
- Positional paresthesias
- Sore leg muscles[14]

Less common conditions include

- Arthritis
- Central or peripheral neuropathy
- Complex regional pain syndrome
- Drug-induced akathisia
- Fibromyalgia
- Leg cramps
- Myopathy
- Sickle cell disease[14]

Several reversible medical diagnoses have shown associations with RLS/WED. These conditions include iron deficiency anemia, vitamin B_{12}/folate deficiency, and pregnancy. Other medical diagnoses associated with RLS/WED include peripheral neuropathy (associated with diabetes mellitus), rheumatoid arthritis, spinal disorders such as spinal nerve root irritation, Parkinson disease, fibromyalgia, chronic and end-stage renal disease, spinocerebellar ataxia (particularly spinocerebellar ataxia type 3), and Charcot-Marie-Tooth disease (type 2).[1,2,13] A more complete list can be found in **Box 2**. A list of the more common causes of secondary RLS/WED can be found in **Box 3**. Additionally, RLS/WED has also been found to be exacerbated by common medications and substances.[2] A list of these more common medications and substances can be found in **Box 4**.

COMPREHENSIVE EXAMINATION FINDINGS

A comprehensive examination is essential for the identification of symptoms consistent with RLS/WED. A detailed subjective examination and an accompanying objective examination, with attention directed toward evaluating the neurologic examination, can rule out other differential diagnoses and assist in a timely diagnosis of RLS/WED.

Subjective Evaluation

A thorough and quality evaluation of patients' family history, psychosocial history, and review of systems can aid in the diagnosis of RLS/WED. Major features of RLS, such as restlessness, akathisia, or sensory misperception in the extremities, occur in other neurologic diseases and may be difficult to disentangle from RLS. Patients do not

---

Box 3
Diseases associated with secondary restless legs syndrome/Willis-Ekbom disease

- Acute spinal cord lesions, stroke, myelitis
- Alcohol abuse
- Amyotrophic lateral sclerosis
- Diabetes
- Excess caffeine, chocolate intake
- Hypoglycemia
- Hypothyroidism
- Iron deficiency anemia
- Lumbosacral radiculopathy
- Multiple sclerosis
- Obesity
- Parkinsonism
- Polyneuropathies
- Pregnancy
- Rheumatoid arthritis
- Spinal stenosis
- Venous insufficiency
- Vitamin deficiencies

Data from Allen RP, Picchietti DL, Garcia-Borreguero D, et al, International Restless Legs Syndrome Study Group. Restless legs syndrome/Willis–Ekbom disease diagnostic criteria: updated International Restless Legs Syndrome Study Group (IRLSSG) consensus criteria–history, rationale, description, and significance. Sleep Med 2014;15(8):860–73; and Nagandla K, De S. Restless legs syndrome: pathophysiology and modern management. Postgrad Med J 2013;89(1053):402–10.

Box 4
Medications associated with the onset of restless legs syndrome/Willis-Ekbom disease

- Alcohol
- Antidopaminergic medications (eg, neuroleptics)
- Antiepileptic medications
- Beta-blockers
- Caffeine
- Diphenhydramine
- Lithium
- Selective serotonin reuptake inhibitors (SSRIs)
- Serotonin-norepinephrine reuptake inhibitors (SNRIs)
- Tricyclic antidepressants (TCAs)

Data from Najmi S, Pourabolghasem S. Restless legs syndrome. Int J Chronic Dis Ther 2015;1(1):1–4.

---

typically report extreme daytime sleepiness or the need for daytime naps as they do with other sleep disorders. However, other sequela of sleep deprivation is present and reported as fatigue, difficulty in concentration, and social and occupational disruptions, leading to a loss of work and social productivity.[1,4,9] Patients frequently report psychological effects and mood disturbances, such as altered mood and depression, anxiety, decrease in short-term memory efficiency, and a worsening health-related quality of life.[1,2,4,6,7,9]

When conducting a review of past medical history, patients often report recurring headaches, snoring with or without obstructive sleep apnea, cardiovascular disease, hypertension, stroke, and signs and symptoms of a hyperactive sympathetic nervous system (eg, dry mouth, constipation or loss of appetite, hyperglycemia, tachycardia).[4] A valuable and predictive finding is a history of other sleep disturbances, such as insomnia, PLMS, obstructive sleep apnea, or snoring.[1] Other reports of vascular disease, such as varicose veins, venous stasis, deep vein thrombosis, or intermittent claudication, have also be reported in greater incidence during interviews with patients who have RLS/WED.[3,13]

During the review of systems, patients are likely to report a wide variety of sensations and experiences. One of the hallmark subjective symptoms is an uncontrollable urge to repeatedly stretch and/or change positions. This urge is typically accompanied by other abnormal sensations variably described as burning, tingling, creepy-crawly or insects crawling under the skin, aching, stretching, pressure, or electrical impulses. All of these sensations are perceived as being inside the legs. The sensations are typically perceived bilaterally and not associated with superficial sensations felt on the surface of the skin.[1] More concretely, patients may report nocturnal leg cramps, deep pains within the muscles, pain in the middle of the lower limbs or calves, pain experienced from movements of the legs or toes (myalgias), arthritis, or general akathisia.[13] Patients report these sensations to be transient rather than continuous, with only partial relief from movement. The pains are worsened by a lack of movement.[1]

Objective Evaluation

With RLS/WED presenting intermittently and predominately occurring at night, limited findings may be discovered during the physical examination. What may be found, however, are the sequelae due to the impact on patients' psychosocial health. These sequelae may include physiologic signs of fatigue, anxiety, depression, decreased quality of life, or sympathetic hyperactivity, such as dilated pupils, dry mouth, hypoactive bowel sounds, hyperglycemia, tachycardia, and elevated blood pressure. The provider should consider using valid and reliable screening tools to either detect RLS/WED or the associated psychosocial outcomes of

- Anxiety
- Depression
- Quality of life
- Fatigue

Outside of the psychosocial findings, the provider may notice volitional movements, such as frequent position changes from discomfort or habitual foot tapping during the subjective questioning or while conducting the physical examination. These findings in isolation are not diagnostic. However, when considering the complete clinical picture, they may provide helpful diagnostic cues.[13]

DIAGNOSTIC CRITERIA

The diagnostic criteria for RLS/WED have continued to be refined and more clearly developed over the past decade. Criteria outlined by the *International Classification of Sleep Disorders*, Third Edition (*ICSD-3*) are similar to those of the IRLSSG.[17,18] The *ICSD-3* criteria differ from those of the IRLSSG in that distress, associated sleep disturbance, or impairment is required to establish the *ICSD-3* diagnosis.[17] This requirement is not the case with the IRLSSG. The diagnosis of RLS using the IRLSSG criteria is made through ascertaining symptom patterns in patients. The patients must meet all 5 essential diagnostic criteria outlined next:

1. An urge to move the legs is usually but not always accompanied by, or thought to be caused by, uncomfortable and unpleasant sensations in the legs.
2. The urge to move the legs and any accompanying unpleasant sensations begin or worsen during periods of rest or inactivity, such as lying down or sitting.
3. The urge to move the legs and any accompanying unpleasant sensations are partially or totally relieved by movement, such as walking or stretching, at least as long as the activity continues.
4. The urge to move the legs and any accompanying unpleasant sensations during rest or inactivity only occur or are worse in the evening or night than during the day.
5. The occurrence of the aforementioned features is not solely accounted for as symptoms primary to another medical or a behavioral condition (eg, myalgia, venous stasis, leg edema, arthritis, leg cramps, positional discomfort, habitual foot tapping).[19]

Several considerations exist within these criteria.

1. When considering criterion 1, the examiner must consider that sometimes the urge to move is present without the uncomfortable sensations and sometimes the arms or other body parts are involved in addition to the legs.[19]
2. For criterion 3, when symptoms are very severe, relief by activity may not be noticeable. However, this must have been previously present.[19]
3. For criterion 4, when symptoms are very severe, the worsening at night may not be noticeable. However, this must have been previously present.[19]
4. For criterion 5, these conditions, often referred to as RLS mimics, have been commonly confused with RLS, particularly in surveys, because they produce symptoms that meet or at least come very close to meeting criteria 1 to 4. The list gives

examples of these that have been noted as particularly significant in epidemiologic studies and clinical practice. RLS may also occur with any of these conditions, but the RLS symptoms will then be more in degree, conditions of expression, or character than those usually occurring as part of the other condition.[19]

5. Patients must answer yes, in their own words, to each question. However, neither a minimum frequency nor duration of events is part of the current diagnostic criteria, as the presence of clinical distress associated with RLS/WED symptoms may vary as to the number of days symptoms are present.[20]

Special attention has been placed on the adaptation and implementation of these criteria to the pediatric population. The Sleep-Wake Work Group of the *Diagnostic and Statistical Manual of Mental Disorders* (*DSM*) Task Force asked for the pediatric RLS criteria to be integrated with the adult criteria before the release of *DSM-5*. It is important to emphasize that if this tool is being used to evaluate children, several standardizations must occur:

- The child must describe RLS symptoms in his or her own words.
- The diagnostician should be aware of the typical words children and adolescents use to describe RLS.
- Language and cognitive development determine the applicability of the RLS diagnostic criteria, rather than age.
- It is not known if the adult specifiers for the clinical course apply to pediatric RLS.
- As in adults, a significant impact on sleep, mood, cognition, and function is found. However, impairment is manifest more often in behavioral and educational domains.
- Simplified and updated research criteria for probable and possible pediatric RLS are available.
- Periodic limb movement disorder may precede the diagnosis of RLS in some cases.[14]

Because the diagnostic criteria require the verbal description of RLS sensations by the child—urge versus discomfort, the relationship of symptoms to rest or inactivity (eg, lying down vs sitting), relief with movement, time of day or night of the occurrence (eg, only or worse at evening/night), and the differentiation from symptoms of other conditions—it is unlikely that most children less than 6 years of age will have the skills to accurately describe their symptoms.[1,14] When attempting to diagnose RLS in the pediatric population, clinical features that support the diagnosis of pediatric RLS are

1. PLMS greater than 5 per hour
2. Family history of RLS among first-degree relatives
3. Family history of PLMS greater than 5 per hour
4. Family history of PLMD among first-degree relatives[14]

In an attempt to streamline the diagnostic process for all individuals, a single standardized question for rapid screening of RLS has been validated by the IRLSSG. This question can be used to effectively screen patients who present with a high suspicion of RLS/WED, as it has shown to have a 100% sensitivity and 96.8% specificity for the diagnosis of RLS:

When you try to relax in the evening or sleep at night, do you ever have unpleasant, restless feelings in your legs that can be relieved by walking or movement?[21]

The use of diagnostic examinations helps to further narrow the differential diagnosis. If a peripheral neuropathy is suspected, an electrophysiologic examination should be considered. Patients with RLS will have normal findings on both electromyography and nerve conduction studies, as RLS/WED is not a condition of nerve conduction or impulse propagation.[13] An overnight polysomnogram may also be used to come to a diagnosis. During this examination, an overnight periodic limb movement index of 5 or more limb movements per hour of sleep is required. However, it is important to remember the diagnosis of PLMS is not diagnostic of RLS. PLMS may occur as a result of sleep-disordered breathing, such as obstructive sleep apnea, or as an adverse drug effect. RLS is not associated with these situations.[4]

TREATMENTS

When considering a treatment plan for RLS/WED, the clinician needs to evaluate the severity and frequency of symptoms when determining a treatment plan. Final treatment plans are more effective when incorporating both pharmacologic (eg, dopaminergic medication, alpha-2-delta calcium channel ligands) and nonpharmacologic (eg, lifestyle changes) interventions. Pharmacologic therapy should be approached with extreme caution and is generally not recommended in pregnancy-related RLS in view of inconsistent reports on the risks of medications to the fetus compared with the relative benign nature of the condition.[4] Patients should also be referred to either a neurologist or sleep specialist if initial treatment plans by a nonspecialist are not successful.[13] The IRLSSG defines unsuccessful treatment as

- There is an insufficient initial response despite adequate duration and dose of treatment; adequate duration depends on the pharmacologic agent being used.
- Response to treatment becomes insufficient despite an increased dose.
- Side effects are intolerable.
- The maximum recommended dosage is no longer effective.
- Augmentation develops.[3]

Augmentation is deemed to be a major side effect related to the long-term treatment of RLS and is most often seen during pharmacologic management with dopaminergic medication. It consists of an iatrogenic increase in the severity of RLS symptoms.[9] A treatment algorithm for RLS/WED can be found in **Fig. 1**.

Pharmacologic Treatment Considerations

Pharmacologic management of RLS may be approached in a variety of ways. Dopamine agonists (eg, pramipexol, ropinirole, rotigotine) or alpha-2 delta calcium channel ligands (eg, gabapentin, pregabalin) have both shown to improve the severity of RLS/WED symptoms.[2,5] A summary of pharmacologic recommendations can be found in **Table 1**. Some initial clinical benefit of fast-acting dopaminergic medications has been seen.[1] In a comparative study, patients with parkinsonism who were not receiving levodopa had higher rates of PLMS when compared with aged patients with parkinsonism who were receiving levodopa.[2,15] These findings help support that dopamine agonists reduce symptoms, at least initially, during dopaminergic treatment.[1] Double-blinded and placebo-controlled studies have also validated the advantages of levodopa and dopamine agonists, such as pergolide, pramipexole, and ropinirole, over other medications.[4] Less evidence is available to support the treatment of RLS/WED with benzodiazepines to aid in quality of sleep or opioid agents in symptoms refractory to first-line treatments, although use of prolonged-release oxycodone/naloxone, methadone, and tramadol has been shown to improve symptom tolerance and increase quality of life in adults who have not responded to other treatments.[4,5,9]

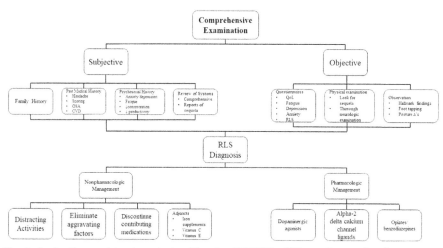

Fig. 1. Evaluation and treatment algorithm for RLS/WED. CVD, cardiovascular disease; OSA, obstructive sleep apnea; QoL, quality of life.

The roles of iron deficiency, iron dysregulation, and brain iron metabolism have not been completely investigated. However, iron supplementation at dosages of 150 to 200 mg/d has been shown to improve iron stores and lessen RLS symptoms. The coadministration of vitamin C and vitamin E can improve absorption of iron, as certain medications, such as proton pump inhibitors, levodopa, and thyroid replacement, can hinder its absorption by the gastrointestinal tract.[2]

Unfortunately, there is no single Food and Drug Administration–approved pharmacologic treatment regimen for pediatric RLS, although studies have shown the efficacy of levodopa and dopaminergic agonists in childhood RLS and associated ADHD.[4] Iron supplementation regimens may be beneficial in the pediatric population when serum ferritin levels are low. Drugs are generally not recommended in pregnancy-related RLS in view of inconsistent reports on their safety and the benign nature of the condition.[4]

Table 1
Pharmacologic approaches to treating restless legs syndrome/Willis-Ekbom disease

Dopaminergic Agents	Dosage
Ropinirole	0.25–4.0 mg daily
Pramipexole	0.125–1.0 mg daily
Rotigotine patch	1–3 mg daily
Carbidopa/levodopa	25/100–200 mg
Alpha-2 Delta Calcium Channel Ligands	**Dosage**
Gabapentin	300–3600 mg daily
Gabapentin enacarbil	600–1200 mg daily
Pregabalin	100–450 mg daily
Adjuncts	**Dosage**
Ferrous sulfate	325 mg BID
Vitamin C	100–200 mg BID
Vitamin E	400 mg daily

Data from Refs.[2,5,9,10]

Nonpharmacologic Treatment Considerations

Nonpharmacologic therapies should be used whenever possible to minimize the risk of drug-on-drug interactions and augmentation, which is a risk of pharmacologic therapies. Initially, the health care provider should assist patients in correcting contributing factors determined from the subjective examination. This correction may include removing unnecessary offending medications known to either cause or exacerbate RLS (eg, selective serotonin reuptake inhibitors, serotonin-norepinephrine reuptake inhibitors, diphenhydramine, dopamine antagonists), modifying the diet to optimize iron consumption, and minimizing caffeine, alcohol, and nicotine intake.[2,3,8,9] Attention should also be directed at lifestyle modifications to increase sleep hygiene measures, implementation of distraction strategies, and development of exercise routines. These lifestyle modifications may represent moderate regular exercise or brief walking and other motor activities with care to avoid overexertion, use of hot or cold baths, whirlpool baths, limb massages, or pneumatic/vibratory/electrical stimulation of the legs, feet, and/or toes through the use of various commercial and medical devices.[2,3,8,9,13]

SUMMARY

RLS/WED is a common sensorimotor disorder characterized by an urge to move and is associated with an uncomfortable sensation typically in the lower extremities. PLMS are seen in 80% to 90% of patients with RLS. However, the presence of PLMS is not diagnostic of RLS/WED. RLS may lead to sleep interruptions and insomnia, resulting in fatigue, depression, decreased quality of life, and significant morbidity.[22] Brain iron deficiency, dopaminergic neurotransmission abnormalities, genetics, sleep deprivation, circadian rhythm disturbances, immobilization, iron deficiency, and/or use of medications that can antagonize dopamine all play key roles in the pathogenesis of primary (idiopathic) RLS, although the exact mechanisms are still unclear. Several associations have also been found with other medical conditions and medication usage for a diagnosis of secondary RLS. Identification and treatment with a thorough subjective evaluation and complete neurologic examination are essential in the diagnosis of RLS/WED. Dopaminergic agents and alpha-2-delta calcium channel ligands are the more common and effective pharmacologic agents used to treat RLS with variable efficacy. Finally, nonpharmacologic treatments are an important adjunct when developing a treatment plan for RLS/WED. Referral to a neurologist or sleep specialist should be considered if initial treatment plans are ineffective or worsen patients' symptoms.

REFERENCES

1. Allen RP, Picchietti DL, Garcia-Borreguero D, et al, International Restless Legs Syndrome Study Group. Restless legs syndrome/Willis–Ekbom disease diagnostic criteria: updated International Restless Legs Syndrome Study Group (IRLSSG) consensus criteria–history, rationale, description, and significance. Sleep Med 2014;15(8):860–73.
2. Bertisch S. In the clinic. Restless legs syndrome. Ann Intern Med 2015;163(9): ITC1–11.
3. Leschziner G, Gringras P. Restless legs syndrome. BMJ 2012;344(2):e3056.
4. Ovallath S, Deepa P. Restless legs syndrome. J Parkinson Dis 2012;2:49–57.
5. Venkateshiah SB, Ioachimescu OC. Restless legs syndrome. Crit Care Clin 2015; 31:459–72.
6. Ohayon MM, O'Hara R, Vitiello MV. Epidemiology of restless legs syndrome: a synthesis of the literature. Sleep Med Rev 2012;16(4):283–95.

7. Nagandla K, De S. Restless legs syndrome: pathophysiology and modern management. Postgrad Med J 2013;89(1053):402–10.
8. Najmi S, Pourabolghasem S. Restless legs syndrome. Int J Chronic Dis Ther 2015;1(1):1–4.
9. Winkelman JW, Armstrong MJ, Allen RP, et al. Practice guideline summary: treatment of restless legs syndrome in adults: report of the guideline development, dissemination, and implementation subcommittee of the American Academy of Neurology. Neurology 2016;87(24):2585–93.
10. Garcia-Borreguero D, Kohnen R, Silber MH, et al. The long-term treatment of restless legs syndrome/Willis–Ekbom disease: evidence-based guidelines and clinical consensus best practice guidance: a report from the International Restless Legs Syndrome Study Group. Sleep Med 2013;14(7):675–84.
11. Aurora RN, Kristo DA, Bista SR, et al. The treatment of restless legs syndrome and periodic limb movement disorder in adults—an update for 2012: practice parameters with an evidence-based systematic review and meta-analyses: an American Academy of Sleep Medicine clinical practice guideline. Sleep 2012; 35(8):1039–62.
12. Understanding possible "mimics" of restless legs syndrome (2016). [PDF document]. Available at: https://www.rls.org/file/mimics-052016.pdf. Accessed December 12, 2017.
13. Klingelhoefer L, Bhattacharya K, Reichmann H. Restless legs syndrome. Clin Med 2016;16(4):379–82.
14. Picchietti DL, Bruni O, de Weerd A, et al, International Restless Legs Syndrome Study Group. Pediatric restless legs syndrome diagnostic criteria: an update by the International Restless Legs Syndrome Study Group. Sleep Med 2013;14(12): 1253–9.
15. Bliwise DL, Trotti LM, Yesavage JA, et al. Periodic leg movements in sleep in elderly patients with Parkinsonism and Alzheimer's disease. Eur J Neurol 2012; 19(6):918–23.
16. Roy M, de Zwaan M, Tuin I, et al. Association between restless legs syndrome and adult ADHD in a German community-based sample. J Atten Disord 2018; 23(3):300–8.
17. American Academy of Sleep Medicine (AASM). International classification of sleep disorders. 3rd edition. Darien (IL): American Academy of Sleep Medicine; 2014.
18. International Restless Legs Syndrome Study Group. Validation of the International Restless Legs Syndrome Study Group rating scale for restless legs syndrome. Sleep Med 2003;4(2):121–32.
19. International Restless Legs Syndrome Study Group 2012 Revised IRLSSG Diagnostic Criteria for RLS. 2012. Available at: http://irlssg.org/diagnostic-criteria/. Accessed December 14, 2017.
20. Ohayon MM, Bagai K, Roberts LW, et al. Refining duration and frequency thresholds of restless legs syndrome diagnosis criteria. Neurology 2016;87(24): 2546–53.
21. Ferri R, Lanuzza B, Cosentino FII, et al. A single question for the rapid screening of restless legs syndrome in the neurological clinical practice. Eur J Neurol 2007; 14(9):1016–21.
22. Li Y, Li Y, Winkelman JW, et al. Prospective study of restless legs syndrome and total and cardiovascular mortality among women. Neurology 2017;90(2):e1–7.

Degenerative or Debilitative Neurologic Syndromes

Abby Luck Parish, DNP, AGPCNP-BC, GNP-BC, FNAP

KEYWORDS

- Neurologic disorders • Dementia • Parkinson disease • Disease presentation
- Treatment

KEY POINTS

- Dementia, the most common neurodegenerative disorder, has several subtypes and is characterized by cognitive and functional decline.
- Parkinson disease is the second most common neurodegenerative disorder and presents with the 3 hallmark motor symptoms of resting tremor, bradykinesia, and rigidity.
- Both dementia and Parkinson disease have significant associated symptoms that warrant assessment and treatment by clinicians.
- Neurodegenerative disorders currently lack effective neuroprotective or disease-mediating therapy; however, some promising therapies are in the pipeline.

The descriptor degenerative is broad, denoting a decline from normal function, typically without a known cause. As health care science has progressed and causes for many neurologic diseases have been discovered, the term degenerative has largely fallen out of favor; however, it may still be used to describe a broad group of disorders characterized by progressively altered neurologic function, ranging from the common (eg, dementia) to the rare (eg, amyotrophic lateral sclerosis [ALS]). This article identifies and describes common neurodegenerative disorders, their diagnosis and management, and current research priorities.

BACKGROUND AND SIGNIFICANCE

In the context of the decline in infectious diseases worldwide with associated increased life expectancy, international public health officials increasingly focus on degenerative diseases or diseases associated with older age, including degenerative neurologic disorders. The World Health Organization (WHO) last updated their report on neurologic disorders in 2006, at which time they estimated that the 2 most common degenerative neurologic disorders, dementia and Parkinson disease (PD), could affect

---

Disclosure Statement: The author has nothing to disclose.
Vanderbilt University School of Nursing, 461 21st Avenue South, Nashville, TN 37240, USA
E-mail address: abby.parish@vanderbilt.edu

as many as 44 million and 7 million persons by 2030, respectively.[1] Neurodegenerative disorders are accompanied by significant disability. The WHO acknowledges this burden, estimating that dementia and PD could result in greater than 17 million years of healthy life lost as a result of disability.[1]

DEMENTIA

The most common degenerative neurologic disorder is dementia. Predominantly a syndrome of older age, there are several known variants of dementia, each of which has a unique pathophysiology, presentation, and trajectory. Despite their differences, each type of dementia causes significant impairments to cognition and function and, at this time, there are no curative therapies available for dementia, regardless of type.

Prevalence of dementia is directly related to age, with older groups being affected in larger numbers (Table 1).[2,3] As of 2010, an estimated 4.7 million Americans older than the age of 65 years had dementia.[2] Overall prevalence is slightly higher in women, which is likely due to women having greater life expectancy than men.[4] Epidemiologic studies predict that as nations become increasingly developed, numbers of persons who are older and thus are affected by dementia will grow, resulting in an anticipated worldwide increase in dementia cases in the coming decades.[4] In addition to advancing age, dementia prevalence is also correlated to a population's overall level of educational attainment and socioeconomic factors. Higher education and socioeconomic status are associated with less obesity and cardiovascular disease, which are known risk factors for vascular and Alzheimer dementia.[4]

Each person with dementia's disease trajectory is unique, with significant individual variation in speed of symptom progression through the cognitive, behavioral, and functional domains. This variation makes it difficult to devise a universal staging schema or tool.[5] However, to capture the typical progression of symptoms, dementia is often conceptualized as having mild, moderate, and severe stages. For most patients, mild dementia is characterized by early deficits in cognition and mild functional deficits.[5] In addition to having progressively worsening cognition and function, persons with moderate dementia often have more frequent and severe behavioral and psychological symptoms of dementia (BPSD).[5] Finally, severe dementia is characterized by advanced cognitive impairment and more vegetative-type symptoms.[5] There is not a standard amount of time spent in each phase; however, those with a generally shorter or more aggressive disease course will often experience shorter periods in the mild, moderate, and severe stages, whereas those with longer disease trajectories may have relatively longer periods in each stage. Persons with dementia have an average of 4 to 8 years from diagnosis to death, though significant variation in survival exists, with some patients surviving 20 or more years after diagnosis.[5]

Table 1 Prevalence of dementia		
Age (y)	Estimated Number of Americans with Dementia in 2010 by Age Group[2]	Percent of Age Group with Dementia[2,3]
65–74	0.7 million	0.032%
75–84	2.3 million	17.7%
85+	1.8 million	34.0%

Types of Dementia

Dementia variants are distinguished by their pathophysiology and thus may be definitively diagnosed on autopsy and examination of neurologic tissues.[6] Differing pathophysiologic changes between dementia variants often results in unique symptoms and disease trajectories, offering clinicians the opportunity to approximate a diagnosis while the patient is living. A description of some of the most common dementia variants and their distinguishing pathophysiologic and clinical features follows.

Alzheimer Disease

Alzheimer disease (AD) is thought to be the most common subtype of dementia. It is characterized by amyloid plaques and neurofibrillary tangles in the cerebrum.[1,6] These plaques and tangles ultimately progress to profound atrophy and shrinking of the brain. Symptomatically, AD most commonly presents with short-term memory loss and difficulty with word finding, and progresses to affect global memory and functioning.

Dementia with Lewy Bodies

Thought to be the second most common type of dementia, dementia with Lewy bodies (DLB) is characterized pathophysiologically by inclusions of alpha-synuclein, known as Lewy bodies, to the amygdala and other regions of the brain.[6,7] Clinically, patients typically present with memory changes, as well as earlier and more prominent visuospatial deficits, visual hallucinations, neuroleptic sensitivity, and (ultimately) Parkinsonian motor symptoms.[7] BPSD are more common in DLB than in AD, leading to a higher utilization and earlier initiation of long-term care in patients with DLB.[8]

Frontotemporal Dementia

A rarer variant of dementia involves frontotemporal cerebral atrophy.[9] Persons with frontotemporal dementia display early social deficits with marked disinhibition, impulsivity, and hyperorality.[9] Frontotemporal dementia typically has an earlier age of onset than other dementia variants, with most affected persons having first symptoms before the age of 65 years.[9]

Vascular Dementia

Vascular dementia is a broad term that is applied to cases wherein a person experiences cognitive deficits after a single vascular event (eg, stroke), multiple cortical infarcts, and/or subcortical cerebrovascular changes.[10] Owing to the variation in pathophysiological changes, significant clinical variation between cases exists and there is not a single vascular dementia phenotype.[10] Vascular factors, such as hypertension, diabetes, and smoking, are known risk factors for the development of vascular dementia of any cause.[10]

Mixed Type

Autopsy studies support the notion that many or even most cases of dementia are multifactorial in nature. For instance, many cases of AD also display evidence of Lewy bodies or impaired vasculature.[6,10] The high suspected prevalence of mixed cases of dementia contributes to the difficulty of accurate diagnosis, and many patients' clinicians will choose a broad diagnosis of dementia or a diagnosis of mixed type dementia rather than a selecting a single type.

Assessment and Diagnosis

A group of experts convened by the Alzheimer's Association established best practice guidelines for clinical assessment and diagnosis of dementia.[11] The panel notes that assessment of cognitive impairment should be an iterative, stepwise process that incorporates formal assessment techniques with collateral information from staff and informal caregivers.[11] Assessment should address both cognitive and functional abilities.[11]

There are many validated tools available for formal screening of cognition, each of which could be useful depending on specific patient and clinic factors. Screening tools may be used either with patients presenting with a memory-related concern or at annual wellness visits.[11] The Alzheimer's Association panel recommends using 1 of 3 tools for initial screening. The recommendation took into account cost, amount of time required for tool use, validation for community setting, and relative freedom from educational, language, or cultural bias.[11] The 3 suggested tools are the Memory Impairment Screen, the General Practitioner Assessment of Cognition, and the Mini-Cog.[11]

Patients who present complaining of symptoms or who have a positive cognitive screen at a routine visit should receive a full dementia evaluation. This workup is often structured over 2 clinic visits to allow ample time for assessment.[11] Evaluation should include a full medical history, comprehensive laboratory work, assessment of multiple domains of cognition and function, neurologic examination, and (possibly) cranial imaging.[11] Workup may occur with a generalist or a specialist in gerontology or neurology.[11]

Currently, there are no broadly accessible laboratory studies or imaging studies to distinguish between types of dementia, so determination of dementia type relies on the careful assessment of symptoms and history by the clinician. This assessment may be difficult, particularly because disease-related changes typically cause patients to be unreliable historians. The most specific means of determining dementia type before autopsy is in-depth neuropsychological testing. Neuropsychological testing may be used at any point in the dementia trajectory to determine specific deficits across domains (eg, visuospatial functioning, executive functioning, language) and to estimate the corresponding best matching dementia types.[12] This testing must be completed by a trained psychologist, requires significant time, and is often cost-prohibitive, therefore many patients rely on their clinician's, who is not a psychologist, best assessment of type.

Treatment

Curative therapy for suspected dementia is not currently available. Instead, treatment goals for dementia include maximizing function, quality of life, mood, safety, and social engagement.[13] Addressing these domains requires a holistic approach that integrates patient and caregiver feedback to develop a comprehensive plan of care. Plans of care must be continually revised to account for disease progression and changing care needs.

Cognitive Symptoms

There are 5 US Food and Drug Administration (FDA)-approved pharmacologic therapies for use in dementia, all of which were developed to preserve cognitive function (**Table 2**). Compounds comprise 2 therapeutic classes: cholinesterase inhibitors and N-methyl-D-aspartate (NMDA) receptor antagonists. Neither class directly addresses the pathologic changes of any of the types of dementia. Instead,

Table 2
US Food and Drug Administration–approved pharmacologic therapies for dementia treatment

Agent	Brand Name	Approved for	Class
Donepezil	Aricept	All stages	Cholinesterase inhibitor
Galantamine	Razadyne	Mild and moderate	Cholinesterase inhibitor
Rivastigmine	Exelon	All stages	Cholinesterase inhibitor
Memantine	Namenda	Moderate and severe	N-methyl-D-aspartate (NMDA) receptor antagonist
Donepezil-memantine	Namzaric	Moderate and severe	Cholinesterase inhibitor or NMDA receptor antagonist

they intend to optimize levels of neurotransmitters that are known to be altered in dementia. Specifically, cholinesterase inhibitors delay the breakdown of acetylcholine[14] and simultaneously block the flow of glutamate through channels of NMDA-receptors.[15]

A recent Cochrane review identified that cholinesterase inhibitors provide persons with AD with small and clinically uncertain benefits.[14] A similar Cochrane review analyzing the class in patients with DLB suggested that patients with DLB may receive a bit more benefit than those with AD.[16] A recent systematic review by Renn and colleagues[17] notes that, because cholinesterase inhibitors are the only available therapy for early or mild dementia, they are very often prescribed to newly diagnosed patients regardless of suspected dementia type, despite a relative paucity of evidence for their efficacy. However, the class has known potential risks, including weight loss, urinary retention, bradycardia, and depression.[17] There is no current consensus on when or if cholinesterase inhibitors should be discontinued as dementia progresses, and the decision to start or continue therapy should be individualized, taking into account patient and family values and preferences.[17]

The last Cochrane review addressing memantine efficacy was published in 2006.[18] It suggested that memantine might have a small beneficial effect, particularly for patients with nonvascular dementia.[18] Similar to cholinesterase inhibitors, uncertainty exists regarding duration of optimal memantine therapy, and individualized assessment and decision-making is advised.

Behavioral and Psychological Symptoms

In addition to cognitive symptoms, persons with dementia experience varying degrees of BPSD, and these symptoms are often prominent enough to warrant treatment. Commonly experienced symptoms include wandering or restlessness, depression, anxiety, apathy, psychosis, agitation or aggression, and socially or sexually inappropriate behaviors.[19] As many as 97% of persons with dementia will experience at least 1 BPSD; some patients will experience many, whereas others will experience relatively few.[19] Behavioral and psychological symptoms are hypothesized to be the result of a combination of factors, including neurobiological changes of disease, untreated acute medical conditions, unmet needs, environmental or caregiver triggers, and underlying psychiatric and/or personality factors.[19]

Nonpharmacological strategies are considered first-line for management of BPSD. Due to the heterogeneity of studies, it is difficult to systematically review and thus to recommend specific techniques that might work for many or most persons with dementia.[19,20] Current recommendations are to personalize interventions with consideration given to patient, caregiver, and environmental factors.[19–21]

If nonpharmacological strategies are attempted and pervasive BPSD persist, pharmacologic strategies may be used. Pharmacologic strategies should particularly be considered when symptoms pose a safety risk to the patient or their caregivers. Although pharmacologic strategies may assist with some BPSD, others are very unlikely to respond to medications, including cognitive symptoms, poor self-care, care refusal, and wandering.[21]

There are no medication classes that have received FDA approval to treat BPSD; however, several classes have been trialed off-label, and these classes are endorsed by clinical practice guidelines for BPSD. Notably, all of the available pharmacologic options have demonstrated only minimal efficacy in trials; therefore, health care providers often use trial and error to find an option that provides a particular patient with benefit for their unique symptoms. Atypical antipsychotics are considered potentially useful for BPSD; however, their benefits must be balanced with potential adverse effects such as anticholinergic effects, metabolic effects, and postural hypotension.[19] Additionally, the class has a FDA black box warning for increased risk of death in persons with dementia.[22] Persons with DLB should avoid antipsychotics due to neuroleptic sensitivity.[19] Other classes of medications that may have marginal effects on BPSD include antidepressants, anticonvulsants, cholinesterase inhibitors, and memantine.[19] Evidence for each of these classes has been limited and results have been mixed.[19] Clinicians may consider trials of these agents in the context of specific symptoms and comorbidities.

Other Considerations

To meet the holistic goals of care for persons with dementia, clinicians may also suggest or provide referral to an array of other services. Patients should be engaged in conversations about decision-making, including living wills, durable power of attorney for health care and/or finances, and end-of-life preferences. Given the progressive nature of dementia, these topics should ideally be raised early in the disease course to give patients the best opportunity to participate and make their wishes known.

More than three-fourths of dementia patients are cared for at home by loved ones, who are known as informal caregivers.[19] Caregiving for a person with dementia is known to be particularly demanding, both physically and mentally, and as many as 23% to 85% of caregivers of persons with dementia are estimated to have depression, which is significantly more than those who are not caregivers.[19] Clinicians can acknowledge and attend to the strain of caregiving by inquiring about caregivers' well-being and needs at each appointment.

Research Priorities

Because current treatment options for dementia do not address underlying pathophysiology of disease, the main research priority for dementia is the discovery of treatments to prevent or halt pathophysiologic changes of dementia. As of 2016, there are 24 agents for dementia in FDA phase III development.[23] Of these, 7 agents are symptomatic therapies similar to existing agents; however, 17 are novel agents aiming to interrupt pathophysiologic changes of dementia.[23] Of the medications aiming to modify disease progression, most target amyloid activity.[23] An example is aducanumab, a human monoclonal antibody that aims to reduce amyloid-β and thus, ultimately, amyloid-related plaques. In FDA phase III trials in persons with mild or prodromal dementia, monthly intravenous infusions of aducanumab have reduced amyloid-β levels with associated clinically significant slowing of decline in dementia symptoms.[24] There are an additional 45 agents in FDA phase II trials and 24 agents in FDA phase I study.[23]

In addition to pharmacotherapy, public health researchers also acknowledge the need for widespread community-based efforts to modify vascular factors that are known to contribute to vascular dementia.[1] Promoting healthy lifestyles through exercise, smoking cessation, and weight modification can reduce the incidence of cerebrovascular disease and other vascular illnesses, and will be an important component of reducing dementia prevalence.[1]

PARKINSON DISEASE

The second most common degenerative neurologic disorder is PD. This syndrome is named for Dr James Parkinson, who first described the disorder in his seminal work, "*An Essay on the Shaking Palsy*," in 1817.[25] Since that original description, significant progress has been made in describing the pathophysiologic underpinnings of disease and in the development of symptomatic therapies. However, similar to dementia, the development of neuroprotective therapies has lagged.

Epidemiologists predict that, by 2040, 770,000 Americans will be affected by PD.[26] Similar to dementia, PD results in debility and lack of function. The WHO estimates that, by 2030, PD will be responsible for 1.35 million years of healthy life lost as a result of disability worldwide.[1] Interestingly, nicotine is protective for the development and expression of PD, and the worldwide reduction in smoking is expected to contribute to a modest increase in the incidence of PD.[26]

The pathophysiology of PD is complex. Primary changes include depigmentation, loss of nerve cells, and gliosis in the substantia nigra. Associated changes include the inclusion of alpha-synuclein Lewy bodies and depletion of dopamine.[25] Current pharmacologic strategies address dopamine depletion; however, notably, this is a later feature of disease. Clinical symptoms of dopamine depletion do not manifest until many years after pathophysiologic changes begin, resulting in a preclinical or masked phase during which significant pathologic change is present and progresses without readily appreciable clinical manifestations.[25,27]

Presentation and Diagnosis

PD was initially classified as a movement disorder and, although there are now numerous known nonmotor symptoms of PD, symptoms that present first and are responsible for most disease-related debility are motor symptoms. The 3 primary motor symptoms of PD are resting tremor, bradykinesia, and rigidity.[28] Symptoms typically begin on 1 side of the body and, throughout the disease course, this leading side of the body experiences new symptoms earlier and to a greater extent than the contralateral side.[28] As motor symptoms progress, the 3 main symptoms of PD combine to create some of the more classically known Parkinsonian traits, including freezing gait, flexed posture, and masked faces.

Nonmotor symptoms of PD are increasingly recognized as being prominent features of disease, affecting both function and quality of life. Autonomic symptoms, including orthostasis and bowel or bladder dysfunction, affect many persons with PD at some point in their disease trajectory.[27,29] Loss of sensation, particularly smell, can occur early in the disease course or even before the onset of motor symptoms.[29] Sleep disorders are strongly associated with PD and can manifest with symptoms that include restless legs, insomnia, rapid eye movement–sleep disorder, and/or excessive daytime somnolence.[27,29] Neuropsychiatric symptoms affect most persons with PD.

Neuropsychiatric symptoms can include depression, anxiety, and psychosis, as well as cognitive impairment.[27,29]

When persons with PD develop cognitive impairment, they are said to have Parkinsonian dementia. About 40% of persons with PD have dementia, which is about 6 times as many as in non-Parkinsonian counterparts.[27] Parkinsonian dementia shares pathophysiologic and clinical features with both DLB and AD.[27]

Persons who present with motor symptoms that can be associated with PD should undergo full evaluation, preferably in a neurology specialty setting. The initial differential diagnosis may include essential tremor; atypical degenerative disorders; such as multiple systems atrophy; and dementias, including AD and DLB.[30] Testing, including olfactory screening and MRI, may support the diagnostic process; however, final diagnosis is based on clinical symptoms and evaluation.[30] A medication trial is often used in the diagnostic process to discern whether symptoms will respond to dopamine correction.[30]

Treatment Options

Treatment of PD is generally categorized as either being for motor symptoms or non-motor symptoms of PD.

Motor Symptoms

Levodopa is the mainstay of PD treatment today. Its use results in the amelioration of all 3 primary motor symptoms of disease.[25] However, levodopa has some notable limitations. First, as symptoms progress, levodopa becomes less effective, both in the degree and duration of its effectiveness.[25,28] The depreciation of duration of action results in what is known as off-time, or periods of the day when motor symptoms reemerge.[28] Additionally, after years of treatment with levodopa, persons may develop bothersome dyskinesias.[28]

In the past 2 decades, an additional therapy for motor symptoms has emerged. Surgical deep brain stimulation of the subthalamic nucleus can result in significant and immediate relief of motor symptoms and drug-related dyskinesias.[31] The procedure is generally reserved for patients who are later in the disease course and have begun to exhaust the benefits of levodopa. Although it may have quality-of-life gains for many patients, surgical-related risks exist, and some studies have reported worsening of some associated symptoms, such as apathy.[32]

Associated Symptoms

The myriad associated symptoms of PD do not generally respond to levodopa and/or deep brain stimulation and thus must be addressed separately. First, clinicians must be attentive to the assessment of associated symptoms throughout the disease course because these symptoms have historically had a tendency to be overlooked.[27] Some symptoms, such as anosmia, do not have known treatment options. However, many common symptoms, such as depression, constipation, and sleep disorders, may be managed with similar therapies as those used in non-Parkinsonian patients.[27]

Research Priorities

Similar to dementia, although symptomatic treatments for PD exist, disease-mediating therapies, typically referred to as neuroprotective therapies, for PD have been more elusive.[25] The dormant phase of PD affords an opportunity to intervene and spare further degeneration if such persons can be identified and treated with neuroprotective therapies. Researchers have begun to analyze the role of alpha-synuclein in the pathophysiology of disease and to consider ways in which manipulation of alpha-synuclein could be conducted to prevent disease progression.[25]

UNCOMMON DEGENERATIVE NEUROLOGIC SYNDROMES

Though uncommon, other degenerative neurologic disorders may be devastating and are thus worthy of brief examination. Due to their particularly harmful effects, these disorders are considered major neurologic research priorities. Many neurodegenerative processes are suspected to share pathologic features with each other, such as mitochondrial dysfunction[33] and oxidative stress.[33,34] Therefore, researchers aiming to target these relatively rare conditions consider both the broad principles of degenerative disease and specific pathologic disease factors.

Spinocerebellar Ataxias

Spinocerebellar ataxias are a group of predominantly hereditary disorders that are characterized by spinal and/or cerebellar dysfunction and ataxia. These typically manifest in childhood or adolescence, affecting an estimated 0.1 to 10 per 100,000 persons.[35] One of the most common variants is Friedreich ataxia, which is an autosomal recessive hereditary ataxia that results from alterations in mitochondrial protein frataxin.[36] Treatment of the dozens of known variants of spinocerebellar ataxia is currently supportive, though novel restorative or preventative therapies continue to receive attention from researchers.[35]

Neuromuscular Disorders

Huntington disease and ALS are examples of profoundly debilitative diseases that belong under the broad umbrella of degenerative neuromuscular disorders. Huntington disease is an autosomal dominant disorder with an average age of symptom onset of 30 to 50 years and an average disease duration of 10 to 25 years characterized by choreatic movements and cognitive degeneration.[37] ALS is a mostly sporadic disorder with an average age of onset of 40 to 70 years, which is characterized by degeneration of muscular function.[38] Although these conditions affect only 30,000 and 20,000 persons, respectively, their profoundly debilitating effects warrant attention and ongoing research.[37,38]

SUMMARY

Researchers have made significant progress in describing the origins and natural history of common and rare neurodegenerative disorders. Alongside these advances, symptomatic therapies for many illnesses have been developed. In the future, neuroprotective or disease-disrupting therapies will be necessary to contain the increasing numbers of affected persons and to spare debility and, ultimately, loss of life.

REFERENCES

1. World Health Organization. Neurological disorders: public health challenges. 2006. Available at: http://www.who.int/mental_health/publications/neurological_disorders_ph_challenges/en/. Accessed January 1, 2018.
2. Hebert LE, Weuve J, Scherr PA, et al. Alzheimer disease in the United States (2010-2050) estimated using the 2010 census. Neurology 2013;80(19):1778–83.
3. U.S. Department of Commerce Economics and Statistics Administration. Age and sex composition: 2010. 2011. Available at: https://www.census.gov/prod/cen2010/briefs/c2010br-03.pdf. Accessed January 1, 2018.

4. Rizzi L, Rosset I, Roriz-Cruz M. Global epidemiology of dementia: Alzheimer's and vascular types. Biomed Res Int 2014;2014:908915.
5. Alzheimer's Association. Stages of alzheimer's. 2017. Available at: https://alz.org/alzheimers_disease_stages_of_alzheimers.asp#overview. Accessed January 1, 2018.
6. Brenowitz WD, Keene CD, Hawes SE, et al. Alzheimer's Disease neuropathologic change, Lewy body disease, and vascular brain injury in clinic- and community-based samples. Neurobiol Aging 2017;53:83–92.
7. McKeith I, Mintzer J, Aarsland D, et al. Dementia with lewy bodies. Lancet Neurol 2004;3(1):19–28.
8. Rongve A, Vossius C, Nore S, et al. Time until nursing home admission in people with mild dementia: comparison of dementia with Lewy bodies and Alzheimer's dementia. Int J Geriatr Psychiatry 2013;29(4):392–8.
9. The Lund and Manchester Groups. Clinical and neuropathological criteria for frontotemporal dementia. J Neurol Neurosurg Psychiatry 1994;57(4):416–8.
10. Perneczky R, Tene O, Attems J, et al. Is the time ripe for new diagnostic criteria of cognitive impairment due to cerebrovascular disease? Consensus report of the International Congress on Vascular Dementia working group. BMC Med 2016;14:162.
11. Cordell CB, Borson S, Boustani M, et al. Alzheimer's Association recommendations for operationalizing the detection of cognitive impairment during the Medicare Wellness Visit in a primary care setting. Alzheimer's Demen 2013;9:141–50.
12. Smits LL, van Harten AC, Pijnenburg YAL, et al. Trajectories of cognitive decline in different types of dementia. Psychol Med 2015;45(5):1051–9.
13. Alzheimer's Association. Management and patient care. 2017. Available at: https://www.alz.org/health-care-professionals/medical-management-patient-care.asp. Accessed January 1, 2018.
14. Birks JS, Chong LY, Grimley Evans J. Rivastigmine for alzheimer's disease. Cochrane Database Syst Rev 2015. [Epub ahead of print].
15. Johnson JW, Kotermanski SE. Mechanism of action of memantine. Curr Opin Pharmacol 2006;6(1):61–7.
16. Rolinski M, Fox C, Maidment I, et al. Cholinesterase inhibitors for dementia with Lewy bodies, Parkinson's disease dementia and cognitive impairment in Parkinson's disease. Cochrane Database Syst Rev 2012;(3):CD006504.
17. Renn BN, Asghar-Ali AA, Thielke S, et al. A systematic review of practice guidelines and recommendations for discontinuation of cholinesterase inhibitors in dementia. Am J Geriatr Psychiatry 2018;26(2):134–47.
18. McShane R, Sastre AA, Minakaran N. Memantine for dementia. The Cochrane Libray 2006.
19. Kales HC, Gitlin LN, Lyketsos CG. Assessment and management of behavioral and psychological symptoms of dementia. BMJ 2015;350:h369.
20. Testad I, Corbett A, Aarsland D, et al. The value of personalized psychosocial interventions to address behavioral and psychological symptoms in people with dementia living in care home settings: a systematic review. Int Psychogeriatr 2014;26(7):1083–98.
21. Kales HC, Gitlin LN, Lyketsos CG. Management of neuropsychiatric symptoms of dementia in clinical settings: Recommendations from a multidisciplinary expert panel. J Am Geriatr Soc 2014;62(4):762–9.
22. Federal Drug and Safety Administration. Postmarket drug safety information for patients and providers. 2008. Available at: https://www.fda.gov/Drugs/DrugSafety/

PostmarketDrugSafetyInformationforPatientsandProviders/ucm124830.htm. Accessed January 1, 2018.

23. Cummings J, Morstorf T, Lee G. Alzheimer's drug-development pipeline: 2016. Alzheimers Demenent (N Y) 2016;2(4):222–32.
24. Sevigny J, Chiao P, Bussiere T, et al. The antibody aducanumab reduces Aβ plaques in Alzheimer's disease. Nature 2016;537:50–6.
25. Fahn S. The 200-year journey of Parkinson disease: reflecting on the past and looking towards the future. Parkinsonism Relat Disord 2018;46(1):S1–5.
26. Rossi A, Berger K, Chen H, et al. Projection of the prevalence of Parkinson's disease in the coming decades: revisited. Mov Disord 2018;33(1):156–9.
27. Chaudhuri KR, Healy DG, Schapira AHV. Non-motor symptoms of Parkinson's disease: diagnosis and management. Lancet Neurol 2006;5(3):235–45.
28. Fahn S. Description of parkinson's disease as a clinical syndrome. Ann N Y Acad Sci 2003;991:1–14.
29. Poewe W. The natural history of Parkinson's disease. J Neurol 2006;253:VII2–6.
30. Tolosa E, Wenning G, Poewe W. The diagnosis of Parkinson's disease. Lancet Neurol 2006;5(1):75–86.
31. Deuschi G, Schade-Brittinger C, Krack P, et al. A randomized trial of deep-brain stimulation for Parkinson's disease. N Engl J Med 2006;355:896–908.
32. Fisher IH, Pall HS, Mitchell RD, et al. Apathy in patients with Parkinson's disease following deep brain stimulation of the subthalamic nucleus. CNS Spectr 2016; 21(3):258–64.
33. Lin MT, Beal MF. Mitochondrial dysfunction and oxidative stress in neurodegenerative diseases. Nature 2006;443:787–95.
34. Barnham KJ, Masters CL, Bush AI. Neurodegenerative diseases and oxidative stress. Nat Rev Drug Discov 2004;3:205–14.
35. Bird TD. Hereditary ataxia overview. GeneReviews 2016.
36. Lupoli F, Vannocci T, Longo G, et al. The role of oxidative stress in Friedrich's ataxia. FEBS Lett 2018;592(5):718–27.
37. Huntington's Disease Society of America. What is huntington's disease. 2017. Available at: http://hdsa.org/what-is-hd/. Accessed January 1, 2018.
38. The ALS Association. What is ALS? 2017. Available at: http://www.alsa.org/about-als/what-is-als.html?. Accessed January 1, 2018.

Paroxysmal Sympathetic Hyperactivity Syndrome Following Traumatic Brain Injury

Elizabeth Compton, RN, MSN, AGACNP-BC

KEYWORDS

- Paroxysmal sympathetic hyperactivity (PSH) • Traumatic brain injury (TBI)
- Sympathetic storming • Autonomic dysfunction

KEY POINTS

- Paroxysmal sympathetic hyperactivity (PSH) is a syndrome defined by the presence of abnormal sympathetic nervous system or motor activity in response to non-nociceptive stimuli, most often observed in the context of severe traumatic brain injuries.
- Although the exact cause of PSH is unknown, a failure to identify and treat this syndrome can result in negative outcomes, such as prolonged hospitalization and/or worse Glasgow Coma Scale score.
- The consensus-based development of the Paroxysmal Sympathetic Hyperactivity Assessment Measure (PSH-AM) tool was a landmark advancement in the assessment and diagnosis of PSH.
- Current treatment approaches focus on pharmacologic management and prevention of specific sympathetic symptoms.
- Future research goals include implementation and validation of the PSH-AM tool, further development of treatment guidelines, and continued research in imaging and patient monitoring to advance theories of pathophysiology.

INTRODUCTION

Although the syndrome of paroxysmal sympathetic hyperactivity (PSH) has been observed for decades in patients with acquired brain injuries, only in recent years has the identification and definition of this condition been simplified in the literature.[1] PSH is a syndrome of episodic sympathetic and/or motor hyperactivity that has paroxysmal occurrence in patients who have an acquired brain injury due to stroke, head trauma, anoxic injury, or other condition, such as hydrocephalus.[2] Although PSH has been observed in the context of conditions like anoxic injury, stroke, hydrocephalus, and infection, it is most frequently observed in the clinical context of traumatic brain injury due to head trauma sustained through a variety of mechanisms including motor vehicle

Disclosures: None.
Division of Trauma and Surgical Critical Care, Vanderbilt University Medical Center, 1161 21st Avenue South MCN D-2106, Nashville, TN 37232-2447, USA
E-mail address: liz.compton@vanderbilt.edu

Nurs Clin N Am 53 (2018) 459–467
https://doi.org/10.1016/j.cnur.2018.05.003
0029-6465/18/© 2018 Elsevier Inc. All rights reserved.

collisions or blunt trauma sustained in an assault or during a fall event. Some of the observed symptoms include tachycardia, fever, increased respiratory rate, diaphoresis, or dystonic posturing (**Table 1**).[1] One factor that has likely contributed to the confusion surrounding this condition involves the nomenclature attributed to this syndrome. In a 2014 search of the evidence, Baguley and colleagues[1] identified more than thirty different clinical terms used to describe the condition and subsequently aimed to standardize the nomenclature associated with this syndrome by narrowing the synonymous terms to *paroxysmal sympathetic hyperactivity*. With a singularly recognized identifier for this syndrome, both existing and future research may be more easily shared, and appropriate treatment more quickly implemented.

PSH after a sustained traumatic brain injury (TBI) has become a priority in clinical research, as case evidence has demonstrated the negative consequences resulting from undiagnosed or untreated cases of PSH.[1] Evidence on the long-term neurologic outcomes of patients with TBIs with PSH based on measures like the Glasgow Outcome Scale has been conflicting; however, this may be due to a failure of outcome measures to capture deficits with adequate sensitivity.[2,3] Future research pursuits may evaluate long-term neurologic outcomes for these patients in order to better define the extent of the impact of PSH. Although impressions gleaned from existing research may be distorted due to inherent study limitations like small sample size, the evidence has consistently indicated that the presence of PSH acts as a risk factor for worse neurologic outcomes in those who have sustained a TBI.[1–7] While the condition has been noted in pediatric patients with brain injuries, this work focuses on the presentation of PSH in the adult population.

INCIDENCE AND CLINICAL SIGNIFICANCE

PSH has also been identified in patients with a variety of neurologic abnormalities, including hydrocephalus and stroke; however, it is most commonly noted in patients who have TBIs.[2] The incidence of PSH in patients with TBIs has ranged from 8% to 33% in existing literature.[3,6,8] The true incidence may be difficult to gauge, however, because of the historical lack of a standardized set of diagnostic criteria for PSH and thus the absence of a standard diagnostic process in the routine management of these patients.

Table 1
Core symptoms of paroxysmal sympathetic hyperactivity by system

System	Abnormal Criteria
General	
Diaphoresis	Presence of mild to severe sweating
Hyperthermia	Body temperature $\geq$37.0°C
Cardiovascular	
Tachycardia	HR $\geq$100 beats per minute
Hypertension	Systolic blood pressure $\geq$140
Respiratory	
Tachypnea	Respiratory rate $\geq$18 breaths per minute
Musculoskeletal	
Posturing	Presence of mild to severe dystonic posturing of extremities

Abbreviation: HR, heart rate.
Data from Baguley IJ, Perkes IE, Fernandez-Ortega JF, et al. Paroxysmal sympathetic hyperactivity after acquired brain injury: consensus on conceptual definition, nomenclature, and diagnostic criteria. J Neurotrauma 2014;31(17):1515–20.

PSH has been more commonly reported in younger adult men; however, this observation may be attributed to the higher proportion of men in the general adult TBI population.[3] Development of PSH after TBI is noted more frequently in patients with more severe brain injuries.[2,3] The evidence also supports that lesions in the midbrain, corpus callosum, and pontine areas of the brain put patients with TBIs at an increased risk of developing PSH, as do lesions in the periventricular white matter and deep gray nuclei.[2] Symptoms of PSH have been noted in patients with TBIs across the hospitalization trajectory from the acute phase within days of the initial injury through post-hospitalization rehabilitation.[2] The presence of PSH episodes may last from a few weeks to several months, and residual dystonia or spasticity has been noted in several cases, though this may not necessarily be a direct result of PSH.[2]

PATHOPHYSIOLOGY

There exist several conjectures on the pathophysiologic basis of PSH syndrome. One of the early theories that has fallen out of favor involves an epileptogenic model that ultimately was not adequately supported by the clinical evidence.[2,8] Existing evidence supports theories based more on the disconnection of cerebral inhibitory pathways from excitatory centers in the cauda of the brain.[2] One theory speculates that the symptoms of PSH result from the disconnection of cortical centers of inhibition from areas of the brain dedicated to maintaining sympathetic tone, such as the hypothalamus or brainstem.[2] The pathways highlighted in this theory, however, fail to explain all of the symptoms that are observed in patients with presumed PSH.[2]

The theory with the strongest evidentiary support is currently known as the excitatory/inhibitory ratio model.[5,6,8,9] This model is described in a process of two parts, with the first involving the disconnection of the inhibitory pathways that originate in the brain and descend to the spinal cord (**Fig. 1**).[2] This abnormal descending signal then leads to an increase in excitatory neuronal activity, which then results in an increase in efferent motor output and sympathetic output at the spinal level.[2] This pathway explains how, in the case of patients with PSH, an action normally considered non-nociceptive like the physical turning of patients would be perceived as nociceptive in the context of impaired inhibitory pathways and overexcited neurons.[2]

Recent research undertakings have included a focus on brain imaging to evaluate lesion locations an attempt to identify patterns and correlations with PSH symptom development, although findings thus far have been inconclusive.[2] Some studies support the theory that scattered lesions or the presence of diffuse axonal injury are linked to PSH development,[2,3] whereas others support the theory that the physiologic burden of localized lesions to the parenchyma of the brain may lead to PSH development.[4,5] One study found a correlation between PSH risk and brain lesions near the midbrain and pontine,[10] whereas another found an association with lesions in the corpus callosum and the posterior limb of the internal capsule of the brain.[11] Additional exploration into neuroimaging with patients with PSH is an area for potential future research, as the volume of neuroimaging studies is limited and findings have been inconsistent.

CLINICAL PRESENTATION

PSH syndrome, particularly after an acquired brain injury, presents as an increase of motor or sympathetic nervous system activity in response to typically benign stimuli that normally would not elicit such a dramatic physiologic response.[2] The clinical features of PSH can include episodes of significant tachycardia, hypertension, diaphoresis, or dystonia that can present suddenly in the absence of a known cause such

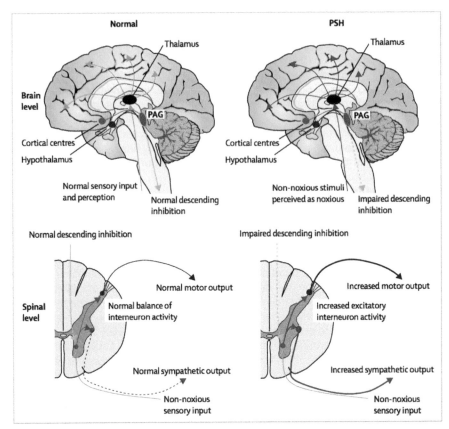

Fig. 1. PSH: theory of excitatory/inhibitory ratio pathogenesis model. PAG, periaqueductal grey. (*From* Meyfroidt G, Baguley IJ, Menon DK. Paroxysmal sympathetic hyperactivity: the storm after acute brain injury. Lancet Neurol 2017;16(9):724; with permission.)

as infection.[1,2] These episodes of sympathetic and motor hyperactivity may individually last from minutes to hours and may occur several times a day.[12] In some publications, severe TBI is defined as an admission Glasgow Coma Score (GCS) of 8 or lower,[5,6,8] although some articles assessed for PSH in patients with a maximum admission GCS of 12.[4,13] The identification and grouping of symptoms present in PSH in the appropriate clinical context have helped better define PSH as a more easily recognizable and diagnosable syndrome.

DIAGNOSIS

Currently, PSH is identified as a diagnosis of exclusion.[1] When evaluating patients in a clinical context, the provider must consider differential diagnoses that could be contributing to the observed clinical presentation. Some of these differential diagnoses include withdrawal from opiates or sedating medications, heterotopic ossification, neuroleptic malignant syndrome, sepsis, or systemic inflammatory response syndrome, to name a few.[1] The lack of a definitive physiologic mechanism has made the standardization of PSH a challenge for clinicians and researchers. In 2014, a panel of experts including many global leaders in PSH research published a consensus-based guideline to identify PSH and classify its severity.[1] Publications until this point included different diagnostic criteria that varied based on factors of clinical assessment, symptom severity, timing of diagnosis, and the number of symptoms required for diagnosis.[2]

The guideline for clinicians established in 2014 by Baguley and colleagues,[1] known as the Paroxysmal Sympathetic Hyperactivity Assessment Measure (PSH-AM) tool, is composed of two parts: the Clinical Feature Scale (CFS) and the Diagnostic Likelihood Tool (DLT) (**Fig. 2**). The CFS component focuses on the severity of symptoms such as elevated body temperature, heart rate, and respiratory rate, and the presence or absence of symptoms like posturing and diaphoresis.[1] Each symptom has categories based on the degree of deviation from physiologic normal and is graded numerically with values increasing with the progression of symptom severity. The CFS total score is a summation of the scores for each symptom, which produces a ranked clinical feature severity score.[1]

The DLT segment of the PSH-AM consists of criteria focusing on the frequency and duration of sympathetic hyperactivity symptoms.[1] If the criteria for a certain category is met, a point is added to the patient's score. The DLT total score is a summation of all of the points within the DLT subsection of the PSH-AM.[1] An overall PSH-AM score is obtained by adding the subtotal CFS and DLT scores. This overall summation score is then used to grade the likelihood of a PSH diagnosis ranging from an "unlikely diagnosis" with scores less than eight, a "possible diagnosis" with a scores ranging from eight to sixteen, and a "probable diagnosis" including scores exceeding seventeen.[1]

The PSH-AM tool, as described by its authors, is intended to be used in a serial fashion, such as daily use at a standardized time in order to assess the trajectory

Clinical Feature Scale (CFS)

	0	1	2	3	Score
Heart rate	<100	100–119	120–139	≥140	
Respiratory rate	<18	18–23	24–29	≥30	
Systolic blood pressure	<140	140–159	160–179	≥180	
Temperature	<37	37.0–37.9	38.0–38.9	≥39.0	
Sweating	Nil	Mild	Moderate	Severe	
Posturing during episodes	Nil	Mild	Moderate	Severe	
			CFS subtotal		

Severity of clinical features	Nil	0	
	Mild	1–6	
	Moderate	7–12	
	Severe	≥13	

Diagnosis Likelihood Tool (DLT)

Clinical features occur simultaneously	
Episodes are paroxysmal in nature	
Sympathetic over-reactivity to normally non-painful stimuli	
Features persist ≥3 consecutive days	
Features persist ≥2 wk postbrain injury	
Features persist despite treatment of alternative differential diagnoses	
Medication administered to decrease sympathetic features	
≥2 episodes daily	
Absence of parasympathetic features during episodes	
Absence of other presumed cause of features	
Antecedent acquired brain injury	
(Score 1 point for each feature present) DLT subtotal	

Combined total (CFS + DLT)	

PSH diagnostic likelihood	Unlikely	<8	
	Possible	8–16	
	Probable	>17	

Fig. 2. PSH-AM. (*From* Baguley IJ, Perkes IE, Fernandez-Ortega JF, et al. Paroxysmal sympathetic hyperactivity after acquired brain injury: consensus on conceptual definition, nomenclature, and diagnostic criteria. J Neurotrauma 2014;31(17):1518; with permission.)

and severity of PSH after an acquired brain injury.[1] Although components of this tool still require formal validation in a clinical setting, the creation of a well-defined set of diagnostic criteria was a significant and progressive step for managing patients with TBI with PSH symptoms. Although the volume of publications using the PSH-AM on target populations is limited, results published thus far have been supportive of its diagnostic strength and promising potential as a tool to monitor PSH management in patients with TBI.[14,15] The long-term implications of a PSH diagnosis after sustaining a severe TBI is not yet clear based on existing research. The authors of the PSH-AM tool recognize that this tool needs formal validation in prospective studies.[1]

TREATMENT

Without a definitive pathophysiologic cause, a standardized PSH treatment approach remains in the developmental stages. The primary aim of treatment is to prevent and address specific sympathetic symptoms. Nonpharmacologic treatment measures should include attempts to minimize symptom triggers as clinically appropriate.[12] Some of these potential symptom triggers can include endotracheal suctioning, turning, or bathing, which unfortunately cannot be avoided in the care of hospitalized patients.[12] Clinicians and family members can minimize triggers by clustering care, anticipating increased PSH symptom severity during bathing, and minimizing unnecessary touching or external stimuli. Additionally, the presence of infection, alcohol or substance withdrawal, or sepsis should be ruled out as potential alternative causes of symptom development when clinically indicated.[12]

The goals of introducing pharmacologic agents include symptom cessation and prevention. Existing pharmacologic interventions focus primarily on symptom-specific treatment and involve several classes of medications used in conjunction, including benzodiazepines, opioids, nonselective beta-blockers, and muscle relaxers (**Table 2**).[3,12] For example, the addition of a beta-blocker to the medication regimen of patients with PSH symptoms can reduce the frequency and severity of the episodes of tachycardia or hypertension. Typically, the most effective approach is concurrent use of several medication types, with medication routes and dosages varying depending on the patients' symptoms and setting.[3] The scheduled daily use of beta-blockers and gabapentin may reduce the frequency and severity of episodes.[3,12] Short-acting medications, such as intravenous beta-blockers and intravenous sedatives, may be used to abort the breakthrough of specific PSH symptoms in the acute care setting.[12] The aim of pharmacologic therapy is to reduce symptom severity and prevent the use of medications that could worsen PSH symptoms, such as dopamine antagonists.[12] Outpatient pharmacologic therapy understandably focuses on symptom management and prevention with oral medications after patients have been transitioned from intravenous therapies.

Secondary brain injuries can occur in the context of persistent symptoms such as uncontrolled hypertension.[12] Uncontrolled or refractory PSH symptoms that are unresponsive to the usual pharmacotherapeutic interventions can also lead to hyperthermia, cardiac damage, and death.[3,12] With close patient monitoring, it may be possible to assess the efficacy of treatment and better understand the continuum of this syndrome over time. The timeline of PSH symptom presence and severity is certainly an area of potential future research as the clinical conceptualization of PSH continues to evolve.

SUMMARY

PSH is a complex episodic syndrome that can significantly impact adult patients with TBIs. Although PSH has been noted in pediatric patients, the literature in that population

Table 2
Common approaches to pharmacologic therapy for paroxysmal sympathetic hyperactivity syndrome

Medication	Mechanism of Action	Target Symptoms	Route: Suggested Initial Dosing	Additional Considerations
Propranolol	Nonselective beta blockade	Hypertension, fever, tachycardia[12]	PO: 10 mg every 6 h (for symptom prevention)[12]; IV: 1–3 mg, may be repeated every 2–5 min (for symptom abortive treatment)[12]	Note that scheduled beta blockade will blunt severity of symptoms
Benzodiazepines	$GABA_A$ agonist	Agitation, tachycardia, hypertension, posturing[12]	Depends on agent used (see following examples): Clonazepam: PO: 0.25–1.0 mg twice daily (for symptom prevention)[12]; Lorazepam: PO: 2–4 mg every 6–8 h (for symptom prevention)[12]; Diazepam: PO: 5–10 mg PO every 8 h (for symptom prevention)[12]; Midazolam IV: 1–2 mg, may repeat every 4 h (for symptom abortive treatment)[12]	May worsen neurologic examination because of sedation[12] (may make it difficult to assess best neurologic examination in patients with brain injuries); Ensure safe medication taper to prevent seizures and worsening PSH symptoms[12]
Opioid	μ-opioid receptor agonist	Tachycardia, allodynic response, pain, hypertension[12]	PO: oxycodone IR, 10–20 mg every 6–8 h (for symptom prevention)[12]; PO: oxycodone ER, 10–20 mg every 12 h (for symptom prevention)[12]; IV: morphine, 2–5 mg, may repeat every 1–2 h (for symptom abortive treatment)[12]; IV: fentanyl, 25–50 mcg, may repeat every 30–60 min (for symptom abortive treatment)[12]	May worsen neurologic examination because of sedation[12] (may make it difficult to assess best neurologic examination in patients with brain injuries)
Dexmedetomidine	Alpha-2 agonist	Agitation, tachycardia, hypertension[12]	IV infusion: 0.2–0.7 mcg/kg/h[12]	Alternative to clonidine when IV agent is required to manage blood pressure, agitation, and heart rate; typically used in ICU setting[12]

(continued on next page)

Table 2
(continued)

Medication	Mechanism of Action	Target Symptoms	Route: Suggested Initial Dosing	Additional Considerations
Clonidine	Alpha-2 agonist	Hypertension, tachycardia[12]	PO: 0.10–0.30 mg every 6–8 h (for symptom prevention)[12] PO: 0.10–0.30 mg PO once (for symptom abortive treatment)[12]	Often used as first-line for hypertension and tachycardia in patients with PSH; does not address all PSH symptoms, so must be a part of multimodal medication regimen[12]
Bromocriptine	Synthetic dopamine agonist	Dystonia, posturing, fever[12]	(give with opiates) initiate 2.5 mg PO every 8 h[12]	Exact mechanism unclear; usefulness reported in combination with morphine[12]
Dantrolene	Calcium ion blocker	Posturing, muscle rigidity[12]	IV: 1.0–2.5 mg/kg, may repeat dose up to maximum cumulative dose of 10 mg/kg/d (then switch to oral dosing)[12]	Risk of hepatotoxicity, recommend monitoring liver function tests[12]
Baclofen	GABA$_B$ agonist	Rigidity, pain, clonus, spasticity[12]	PO: 5 mg every 8 h, titrate to maximum of 80 mg/d[2] Intrathecal baclofen: will need surgical consult for administration[12]	Risk of cerebral spinal fluid leak with the use of intrathecal baclofen[12]
Gabapentin	GABA agonist	Spasticity, pain, agitation[12]	PO: 100 mg every 8 h[12]	Has some sedative properties, may contribute to improved agitation[12]

Abbreviations: ER, extended release; GABA, γ-aminobutyric acid; h, hours; ICU, intensive care unit; IR, immediate release; IV, intravenous; PO, per os.

Data from Samuel S, Allison TA, Lee K, et al. Pharmacologic management of paroxysmal sympathetic hyperactivity after brain injury. J Neurosci Nurs 2016;48(2):82–9.

is limited. Failure to recognize and address this disorder can have negative implications on the trajectory of patient recovery. Though the exact physiologic origins of this disorder are not explicit, research findings have aided in the definition and understanding of PSH as a condition. Although the establishment of PSH diagnostic criteria by expert consensus was a breakthrough for the approach to clinical recognition and management of PSH, the PSH-AM has limitations and still requires prospective research and validation as a diagnostic tool. Treatment is focused primarily on symptom management and prevention and oftentimes is patient-specific and assessment-oriented. PSH is an important differential diagnosis to consider in patients with severe TBIs due to the risk for worse outcomes if PSH is not recognized and addressed.

REFERENCES

1. Baguley IJ, Perkes IE, Fernandez-Ortega JF, et al. Paroxysmal sympathetic hyperactivity after acquired brain injury: consensus on conceptual definition, nomenclature, and diagnostic criteria. J Neurotrauma 2014;31(17):1515–20.
2. Meyfroidt G, Baguley IJ, Menon DK. Paroxysmal sympathetic hyperactivity: the storm after acute brain injury. Lancet Neurol 2017;16(9):721–9.
3. Choi HA, Jeon SB, Samuel S, et al. Paroxysmal sympathetic hyperactivity after acute brain injury. Curr Neurol Neurosci Rep 2013;13(8):370.
4. Baguley IJ, Slewa-Younan S, Heriseanu RE, et al. The incidence of dysautonomia and its relationship with autonomic arousal following traumatic brain injury. Brain Inj 2007;21(11):1175–81.
5. Fernandez-Ortega JF, Prieto-Palomino MA, Garcia-Caballero M, et al. Paroxysmal sympathetic hyperactivity after traumatic brain injury: clinical and prognostic implications. J Neurotrauma 2012;29(7):1364–70.
6. Mathew MJ, Deepika A, Shukla D, et al. Paroxysmal sympathetic hyperactivity in severe traumatic brain injury. Acta Neurochir (Wien) 2016;158(11):2047–52.
7. Dolce G, Quintieri M, Leto E, et al. Dysautonomia and clinical outcome in vegetative state. J Neurotrauma 2008;25:1079–82.
8. Hendricks HT, Heeren AH, Vos PE. Dysautonomia after severe traumatic brain injury. Eur J Neurol 2010;17(9):1172–7.
9. Perkes I, Baguley IJ, Nott MT, et al. A review of paroxysmal sympathetic hyperactivity after acquired brain injury. Ann Neurol 2010;68(2):126–35.
10. Lv LQ, Hou LJ, Yu MK, et al. Prognostic influence and magnetic resonance imaging findings in paroxysmal sympathetic hyperactivity after severe traumatic brain injury. J Neurotrauma 2010;27(11):1945–50.
11. Hinson HE, Puybasset L, Weiss N, et al. Neuroanatomical basis of paroxysmal sympathetic hyperactivity: a diffusion tensor imaging analysis. Brain Inj 2015; 29(4):455–61.
12. Samuel S, Allison TA, Lee K, et al. Pharmacologic management of paroxysmal sympathetic hyperactivity after brain injury. J Neurosci Nurs 2016;48(2):82–9.
13. Lv LQ, Hou LJ, Yu MK, et al. Risk factors related to dysautonomia after severe traumatic brain injury. J Trauma 2011;71(3):538–42.
14. Monteiro FB, Fonseca RC, Mendes R. Paroxysmal sympathetic hyperactivity: an old but unrecognized condition. Eur J Case Rep Intern Med 2017. Available at: https://ejcrim.com/index.php/EJCRIM/article/view/562/663. Accessed October 26, 2017.
15. Godo S, Irino S, Nakagawa A, et al. Diagnosis and management of patients with paroxysmal sympathetic hyperactivity following acute brain injuries using a consensus-based diagnostic tool: a single institutional case series. Tohoku J Exp Med 2017;243(1):11–8.

Moving?

Make sure your subscription moves with you!

To notify us of your new address, find your **Clinics Account Number** (located on your mailing label above your name), and contact customer service at:

Email: journalscustomerservice-usa@elsevier.com

800-654-2452 (subscribers in the U.S. & Canada)
314-447-8871 (subscribers outside of the U.S. & Canada)

Fax number: 314-447-8029

Elsevier Health Sciences Division
Subscription Customer Service
3251 Riverport Lane
Maryland Heights, MO 63043

*To ensure uninterrupted delivery of your subscription, please notify us at least 4 weeks in advance of move.